PRAISE FOR BIGGER LIVING, SMALLER SPACE

"Reading Bigger Living, Smaller Space is like stepping into the home you always wanted to live in: it's warm, welcoming, comfortable, cozy AF, as vibrant as it is functional, and a real breath of fresh air. Judy Granlee-Gates is the friend we all need to hold our hand through the challenging but oh-so-rewarding work of decluttering and resizing: equal parts blunt, tough-love coach and understanding bestie. If you want to love where you live and easily lay hands on what you actually use, but don't go in for spartan minimalism, Bigger Living, Smaller Space is the user-friendly, no-nonsense guide you've been waiting for."

— ADRIENNE MACIAIN PH.D., AUTHOR
OF *SPARK GENIUS* & *RELEASE YOUR
MASTERPIECE*

As Judy outlines in her book, there are so many benefits to decluttering and resizing.

For years I was constantly losing important papers and replacing items I couldn't find. And I dreaded the thought of anyone dropping by unannounced due to the clutter in my home. Getting help and implementing a new mindset and habits allowed me to create a home and workspace that is warm and welcoming.

Take the first step towards a tidier, more harmonious home by reading this book. With its helpful tips and tough love approach, you'll learn how to tackle the clutter and transform your space into a more productive and inviting environment.

— LYDIA MARTIN, DIGITAL SYSTEMS COACH &
LAUNCH STRATEGIST

Judy is a question asking, problem solving, and insightful friend who shares truth and wisdom with compassion and empathy.

A perfect blend of exploring the joy and freedom that decluttering will bring, to your head, heart and home. You'll be inspired, challenged and grateful for Judy's practical and simple tips for exploring what your life might look like without an excess of clutter around you.

— AMY REVELL, HOST OF THE ART OF
DECLUTTERING PODCAST

I never considered that decluttering could be so beneficial to other aspects of life or be so mindful. I did not know I needed *"Bigger Living, Smaller Spaces"* or to declutter until I read this. It is well written and the author is easily relatable, giving great examples from her own life. Most importantly is that it delves into the why's, while still giving you thought-provoking helpful hints. As an attorney that helps my clients with some of the most stressful times in their lives, I believe this book is a great aid for positive change and highly recommend it for everyone who wants to live "Bigger".

— RENA MCDONALD, ESQ., MCDONALD LAW
GROUP, LLC

Unlike other books on decluttering, Granlee-Gates' charming, refreshing, no-nonsense approach will inspire you to embrace simple living to create a freer, more abundant life. Highly recommended!

— MIMI RICH, MA, LICENSED MARRIAGE AND
FAMILY THERAPIST

What a beautifully thoughtful and insightful book on a not very sexy topic, decluttering. Through magical storytelling Judy gets to the heart of WHY it is important to live with less. Perfectly laid out and easily digestible Judy makes decluttering and organizing fun. If you want to have a richer, fuller life I encourage you to read this personal development book that reads more like your cool aunt's memoir on what's really important. Loved it!

— JESSICA BUTTS-PSYCHOTHERAPIST, AUTHOR,
MYERS BRIGGS TRAINER AND MINIMALIST

Reading Judy's book came at the best time for me as I am helping clients and family members look at what they have amassed over the last several decades. Her simple, no-nonsense approach is practical with a kind delivery. She validates how so much of a right-sizing or resizing process is fraught with emotional landmines! I will incorporate the 4 G's now and forever with Judy's voice guiding me along the way. A book for all!!

— RYAN LANIER, AUTHOR AND ORGANIZING
COACH

BIGGER LIVING, SMALLER SPACE

Resizing for a Clean & Cozy Home

JUDY GRANLEE-GATES

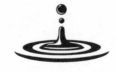

Red Thread Publishing LLC. 2023

Write to info@redthreadbooks.com if you are interested in publishing with Red Thread Publishing. Learn more about publications or foreign rights acquisitions of our catalog of books: www.redthreadbooks.com

Paperback ISBN: 9781955683432

Ebook ISBN: 9781955683449

Cover Design: Sierra Melcher

Author Photo© Emma Nicole

In 1993, I was gifted a tiny microcassette recorder by a dear friend so I could capture ideas and thoughts for my book anywhere, anytime. It only took 30 years to make it happen. Thank you Nancy Buhrman Balduf for the gift of your friendship, love and laughter for so many years. You believed in me more than I believed in myself, and I miss you every single day.

CONTENTS

PREFACE

I began my own decluttering process after inheriting so many possessions from my relatives when they passed away. In my spacious home, all the closets, nooks and crannies were full, and even though the spaces were well organized, the stuff wasn't all useful. Many items were just being kept because I didn't know what else to do with them. Furs, china, silver services: too valuable to just toss, but no real need or market for them, so they stayed.

Shortly after realizing all these things had to at least be sorted through, the idea of resizing registered in a real way for me. Our daughter was getting ready to go to college, and we lived in a large home that we were not using fully. Could building a smaller, more compact home that met all our needs lead us to simpler living? Less stuff, more time to enjoy ourselves?

What if I was wrong? I knew I would have to declutter fully to resize. So, after helping so many others transform their living spaces, my husband and I agreed it was time for us to give it a shot.

For our family, resizing has been a major gift. The gift of more time, freedom, and funds for other things. We love our little house so much, and I know that, for many, the feeling of freedom after this process is so rewarding.

So, what is resizing? It's an adjustment of your home life, much like downsizing, but more tailored to your specific needs. You may resize to a smaller home, the same size home, or any number of other options. Resizing is about adjusting the scale of your home to fit the needs of your current lifestyle and phase. Everyone's choices will be different, including many who just want to declutter, which still resizes your space!

I am a custom builder and remodeler of 34 years to date, and I hear the craziest things when people come in to discuss building or remodeling a home. I recall one couple who insisted they wanted a huge basement game room and second kitchen, because sports events and entertainment were high on their priority list. However, their budget was about $100k lower than they needed to make that happen. In the end, they chose not to build, unwilling to adjust the home plans to fulfill their wishes another way, by enlarging the main living area and kitchen slightly to accommodate the same setup, without a separate space.

Only in America! "I can't have everything I want, so I'm not doing it." I see this often.

In my work, I have met with several thousand people wanting to build or remodel. I have seen some homes so cluttered you could hardly walk in, and the owners felt that adding a little more space or reconfiguring their kitchen would fix their problems. More space is not usually the answer.

I am a professional problem solver. That is how I spend each and every day, regardless of where I am or what my role is. Solving problems from minor to major. Recently, a new friend told me I had an "incredible talent for encouraging." I had never really thought of it that way, but what a compliment! Over the years, I have helped and encouraged people to declutter their homes, often followed by a resizing move so they can enjoy where they live and free up physical, mental and financial energy to live a richer, fuller life.

My home is my sanctuary. My hidey-hole, a term I love from my friend Carrie. The place I recharge and reset, and I can't do that in a place of chaos. It must function, but also have a peaceful and cozy vibe.

I love a beautiful, color-filled, and visually entertaining space. It has a positive mental and emotional impact on me.

I wrote this book to share what I have learned and created, as a guide to get others to a better place in their homes. Your home doesn't have to look and act like mine, it needs to fit *you*. I hope this book will help you define and create that space with the steps, input, and tools I have gathered to live a life that is richer in experience and memories than just managing stuff.

Before we get too far, I will let you know that I am a bit of a tough-love coach when it comes to decluttering and resizing. There is no substitute for hard work, and this process requires that for most to be successful. I am a results-driven person in most everything I do, and you may at times think, "Wow, she is being a little bossy." I am, I admit it. And the reason is, from my own personal experiences, some tough love is required in many cases. By me, and by you!

Before writing this book, I did some research, but maybe not the kind you would think. I didn't read other authors' books on the subject, or check out podcasts and shows. I read book reviews, and really only the 1-, 2-, and 3-star ones. Every single book review that was average or low was fascinating to me; they all said mostly the same thing: "No new ideas." "No new tips to help me." "Nothing new in this book to get me on track."

What I really read was: "I was not willing to do what the author suggested, and thereby, had no results." Yet countless reviewers blamed their lack of action on limited new information. I am here to tell you that the decluttering process is very labor-intensive. It takes *effort*. Thought. Decision making. Dealing with feelings. Not stuff most folks enjoy, but all required components to be successful at pretty much anything in life.

My research confirmed something I have always believed: that there really are no original ideas. No magic bullets. I can simplify it this way: if you have 20 pounds to lose, it's going to take work, exercise, and eating right. In other words: shutting your pie hole (ouch, more tough love!). The same applies here: no magic formula; effort is required to see results.

Years ago I saw a quote that changed my mind about many things. I had often told myself I lacked the ability to follow through on specific tasks. It was my loophole. Then one day, I read this:

"If you are tired of starting over, stop quitting" -Autumn Calabrese.

That got my attention, and I reminded myself of this quote every time I lost focus. I have stopped quitting, and it has led me to a place of achievement and happiness, proving that I don't actually lack focus or follow through. I have used this mindset trick to lose weight, maintain an exercise routine, get my house in order, and more.

Studies and surveys show that clutter alone causes mental health issues, weight gain, increased stress, and more housework.

My hope for you is that you find some nuggets of truth in these pages that light you up and inspire change. I suggest a full read-through first, to absorb the information and concepts, prior to your own declutter and maybe even resize. Using the action steps at the end of each chapter will help you create the path to what works best for you and your family.

For more information about Bigger Living, Smaller Spaces, speaking, podcast appearances or book club opportunities, as well as all things decluttering and resizing, visit my website at www.judygranlee-gates.com.

Chapter One

BIGGER LIVING, SMALLER SPACE IS THE NEW BLACK

*W*ho is this book for, and how do I use it?

Well, there are several types of people this book is for. There are the people living in a bit of a chaotic environment, who have a little too much stuff and are not able to manage it well, find things, have friends over, or who are just spending too much time and energy on their possessions!

The next group is considering resizing their home. The two do go hand in hand, but there is a lot to think about before you resize. Decluttering is a must for resizing, otherwise you have 10 pounds of shit in a 5 pound bag. Since you're reading this book, you're probably interested, but maybe you still have some fear or trepidation around diving in.

There is, however, a group of people that my book is NOT for. Hoarding, defined by a persistent fear or discomfort around the very idea of parting with possessions, regardless of their actual value, is a bonafide mental illness. I'm not qualified to tackle that issue, and would encourage anyone facing this challenge to get help from a team of professionals skilled in that area.

The first way to use this book is just to get an overview of the decluttering and resizing process, before you decide whether either process is for you.

The second way people might use it is as a guide to simply declutter. Decluttering is a major process that can be overwhelming, and is much easier when broken into simple, manageable, and actionable steps. I will lay that out for you here. And if "all" you do is declutter, *you go!* That in itself is a significant process, and it will change how you live in your home and impact your quality of life significantly.

The last way the book might be used is as a step-by-step guide to resizing and living smaller from mindset, to sorting, to processing. Smaller living is on the rise for so many reasons. I hope this book will help you see if it is for you!

Grab a notebook and section it out by the chapters in this book. I suggest you read the entire book first, before starting your process. As you go, make note of things that apply to your situation, any blocks or struggles you have, thoughts on special items, etc., so that you can keep track. You may even see some patterns emerge that can help you move forward.

Before we really dive in, I'll ask you to think about a few things, and to ask yourself some hard questions. You will need to make some time and space to do that and really give it attention or even a family discussion.

- Do you just want to resize your possessions, or do you really want to resize your home, too? This may come later: a thorough declutter can completely transform how you feel about the space you are living in.
- What do you require in a home in terms of space? What rooms *must* you have? Do you really need a dining room, or do you need office space? Can your laundry room be combined with another space? Think carefully about the rooms in your home you actively use, and those you don't. Or those you just stuff crap in and close the door.
- Can you test the smaller living theory out before making a major change? Perhaps you could go on a vacation, live in a smaller space via Airbnb or Vrbo and pretend it's real

life. How does it feel? Will it work for you? Would you need more, or less space?

- Can you remodel your current home to be more efficient? It's amazing what you can accomplish, the space you can create, with the right design. If you love your area or neighborhood, stay where you are. You can also create rentable space that allows you to stay put and rent out a space like an efficiency apartment or even a room on Airbnb, to allow for income generation.
- Is building a home from scratch a good idea for you? After building 800 homes (so far) I can tell you: custom building is so fun, and you get exactly what you want! But that vision is challenging for some, and honestly, we are in times where building is a more expensive option in most areas than buying a resale home. Consider all those options, including buying a resale home that you can remodel if needed.
- What can you compromise to get what you want and need? The family that wanted the big basement game room and kitchen never built their dream home because if they couldn't have everything just the way they envisioned it, they didn't want to do anything at all. To me, that's sad. There are so many ways to get to the finish line of your goals using the tools available to you. Be creative!
- Prioritize. What do you want and need? What are your top three deal breakers? An amazing kitchen, hardwood floors, a craft room? Talk it out and make the list. Where can you compromise? Do you want a luxurious tub? Can it be in any bathroom, or does it have to be in the primary bath? Can any rooms do double duty? Can the guest room have a Murphy bed and double up as a home office and your gym (spoiler alert: it can, and it will be amazing). Think a little bit outside the box, make the list of spaces you need, and think about how some could be combined.
- Can the kids share a room? You know, for decades, they did, and they mostly turned out fine. The key is really in making sure that each kid has their own space, which is doable. A

slightly larger room makes a great shared space, and there are many ways to create privacy, work areas and the rest in rooms that are shared by siblings, especially if they are the same gender.

- If it's just you, start this process of making lists and asking yourself the hard questions. If you have a spouse, partner, or other family members, work together as appropriate to create a blueprint for your family that you can begin to build on.

If you answered yes to more than half of these simple questions, I think you are in the right place, and ready for a change.

CHAPTER ACTION STEPS:

1. *What do you need in your home to make it more functional?*
2. *Do you just need decluttering, or do you have a bigger goal (now or in the future) to resize?*
3. *Make a list of the spaces and areas you need in a home. Can your existing home accommodate you, or is looking at other options or a remodel in your future?*

Chapter Two

LITTLE GHOSTS AND THEIR INCREDIBLY LOUD VOICES

I am the granddaughter of Fran Nelson.
Fran was the undisputed matriarch of the Nelson family, and when she spoke, people listened carefully. Fran was the keeper of all things that came before her. She told me stories of her childhood and youth, and my ancestors I never met. She taught me about sentimentality, the importance of family values, and that being active in your community was a duty, not just something you did if you had time. She was an amazing woman who lived into her early 90s. She valued tough love before anyone knew the term. And when she passed away, the mantle of family historian and keeper of all things Nelson and other families as they married in, fell to me to carry on. My deep love for her kept me wanting to uphold this responsibility, and I treasured all the things that had been left behind.

In 2014 I had come out of a 10-year period where I lost 15 very, very special people. That had been a hard 10 years. Losing both my parents, both my maternal and paternal grandmothers, my husband's grandmother, my father-in-law, two cherished friends, and many others. As each left this life, possessions were left behind, and even as I tried carefully to not over-commit to the many things, I ended up with a lot of "new-to-me" possessions.

I stashed these inherited goods accordingly throughout my house: under beds, in closets, in storage bins. Pretty much all over the place. I had so much stuff, I didn't really know what I had. But it hadn't yet reached a crisis level. My house was neat and tidy, I could still open a closet door without an avalanche hitting me, but I often couldn't easily lay hands on what I wanted. I knew I had seen it, but where? I realized at some point that I would have to sort through all these things and figure out what to do with them.

One dreary early spring day, I wandered into my spacious walk-in closet, and I could just feel a negative energy. I'd inherited many of my mom's collections of beautiful things—lots of jewelry, etc.—and much of it was in easy visual range when I would walk into my closet daily.

One day it occurred to me that all these things were just little ghosts. Little ghosts that reminded me at each glance that these people were no longer here. Little ghosts that tugged at my heartstrings when I needed to be focusing elsewhere. And little ghosts that just left me feeling generally sad.

I reflected on it all day. Couldn't figure out what the heavy feeling was. And then I realized there were the ashes of five dead people in my closet. Mind you, not all the ashes of each person, but somehow, I had a bag of ashes for 5 relatives. My Nana, my grandma, my mom, my dad and my beloved Uncle John. Their ashes, all in boxes on the floor, behind fancy clothes I only wore for special occasions.

I recalled my Uncle John telling me before his death from cancer, that he wanted to be cremated so that his ashes could be scattered in the places he loved all over the world. So, I took the next day off. I loaded up all five of my favorite relatives' ashes in my car, cranked up the tunes, and headed an hour and a half west to make the first stop. There I sprinkled my beloved Grandpa Bob on the site of his old boat yard on Ediz Hook, and my dad, too, since his coast guard base was just a few hundred feet past the boat yard.

This went on all day. Varying stops at beaches, mountains and other places in a three-hour radius from my home, spreading the ashes of each relative, and sometimes more than one. By the end of the day, all five of my relatives had been set free into the universe in places that they loved and were special to them.

The next day, there was a lightness I can't describe, and a shift in my outlook. I decided that the little ghosts needed to be evicted as well. I walked through the house with a small box and picked up all the precious and pretty little things that I enjoyed but really didn't have a lot of use for. I didn't wear them. I didn't use them. And most of them just served as reminders that these people were physically gone from my everyday life. So, I packed them all up and wrote notes to friends of my mom's, and friends of mine who knew her, and I mailed them out one by one with messages telling them how my mom would want these things being worn, used, and enjoyed in the hands of people who were special to her, not just sitting around.

I got a lot of replies. People were thrilled to have received something so personal. It also helped me feel better about sharing her things instead of just keeping them because they were special to her but not to me.

This set me on a journey of really looking at what was in my house. Our daughter was a junior in high school, soon to be graduating and off to college, and I knew that, when she left, my husband and I would be roaming around this big house by ourselves, really living only on one of the three floors.

It seemed silly for us to stay in such a big house. We were paying a gardener, a housekeeper, maintenance people, significant property taxes, a decent mortgage payment each month, insurance, and higher heating and utility bills.

I thought about my grandparents before me, who had resized to move to an apartment when their home got unmanageable. And then to assisted living, and ultimately to nursing care. I realized that, one day, all these lovely things that had been bestowed to me in similar circumstances would in turn need to be bestowed to someone else. Either on my own or by force. By force didn't sound fun. I'd been there too many times before. Several grandparents, other family members, friends' family members. I've assisted with at least half a dozen if not more major life transitions. Sometimes more than once for the same family member.

It gave me the idea that possessions needed to be managed more carefully. Just like money and health. And we had also just come out of a major recession. And so, the costs of living and how the world was changing were on my mind as well.

One day, I woke up and wondered if maybe we should resize NOW, in our early 50's. That would be interesting. Could we live in a small house? I was unsure, but that is how we started out in life, and we were really happy. Could we go back there? I didn't know.

I hatched a plan. Over the next year, I would go through every room, closet, under each bed, every cabinet and drawer, box, and shelf in my house. Even the garage, and *gasp* all my husband's stuff too. I would systematically get rid of the things that didn't bring me/us some pleasure, were useful or necessary. They didn't have to "spark joy" like Marie Kondo says (a toilet brush hardly sparks joy, but you need it, right?), but they did have to hold some special value or, at a minimum, usefulness, to be allowed to stay. And so, it began.

I'm not a professional organizer. I am 100% NOT a minimalist. Not a therapist. I'm none of those things. I do like organization, I am good at it, and I am highly skilled at creating and executing a plan.

I was raised by a neat freak whose home always looked like it was ready for a House Beautiful Magazine photoshoot. In the mid-1970's we had Carrara marble countertops and carpets in the kitchen and baths of our upper middle-class home. My daily chores after school included snapping the rake attachment on the 200-pound Kirby vacuum and then perfectly vacuuming each row of carpet to create symmetrical lines. Some days we just raked; we had 3-inch long multi-color green shag carpets. They were hideous, but when properly raked, they looked lovely for about 3.2 seconds. We were not allowed to make Kool aid or Jell-O in the kitchen, as it might stain the counters.

When I left home, I tossed clothes on the floor, piled dishes in the sink and more as sort of a personal rebellion. As I aged though, my upbringing caught up with me and I too wanted a beautiful tidy space.

I enjoy beautiful spaces. I love sitting on my couch just enjoying the home environment I have created. Creating a rich homelife is an art. It feels like me, and I love spending time there. I prefer form over function, I must admit. I like function, but it has to look good. I understand that not everyone feels that way, but since we have just "met," I thought I would share that since I'll be talking a lot about my style and what I prefer. You may prefer something different, functional may be all you need and want, and that is great. Take what works, and leave the rest.

At the time of this writing, we are 2.5 years into a global pandemic of the COVID-19 virus. It seems to be turning to an endemic, but ever-so-slowly. The last few years have been like no other for most folks: spending a lot of time at home, cooped up with all their family members. Going from working in an office to most everyone working from home, at least for the time being.

These changes really got people looking at their homes in a new light, and wanting their home to function better, look better, and feel better. It honestly did launch a wave of home improvement, both by professionals and DIYers. Many people shifted their view of their home from being simply shelter to being a warm and welcoming environment. And they needed new spaces for things like work and school, and more than one location.

Even as we transition to a post-pandemic world, many people will continue working remotely, and people's homes will continue to shift and change to create more balance now that their work life and home life are so closely intertwined.

I am a firm believer that any space you spend a lot of time in should feel welcoming, warm, and be a place that allows you to reset and recharge. As a remodeler, I often remind people that a huge part of remodeling is not just to prepare a home for sale, but an investment in your environment that will pay off when you go to sell. Enjoying my home, for me, is crucial to my overall happiness.

In the last few years, housing, and the cost of living in general, have spiraled out of control. The unhoused population is growing at an alarming rate. So many people where I live can't afford to live here any longer because rents and sales prices are so high, and the cost of living has not kept up. Every day, I see another family living in their van, and I am not in a major metro area. I see people online asking for help and resources, and people lamenting that they "must" look at smaller homes to rent that they can afford (hopefully), even though their kids will have to share a bedroom. Older residents can no longer afford their paid-off home because the taxes and insurance are like a mortgage payment. If they sell, they must go elsewhere since there is nothing they can afford here.

As a builder/remodeler, I hear talk of "affordable housing" and I am sorry to say that is a thing of the past. We can't build affordable housing when the building code requires an electric vehicle charger in every home with a garage, regardless of the owner wanting it or even having an electric car. Road impact fees of $4500 per home permit, school impact fees in some areas of $4200 per home. Permits alone cost about $12,000 on average for a medium-priced home where I live in Western Washington State.[1]

CHAPTER ACTION STEPS:

1. *Read on with an open mind. Many of the concepts can easily be shrugged off as "not for me." Hold space for new ideas and see what comes up.*
2. *I suggest reading the entire book before taking any action, then revisiting areas as needed. Make notes in the margins and highlight the stuff you want to easily recall.*
3. *Make notes as you go. Feelings that pop up and feel like resistance, ideas you like, areas you know you will have trouble with. These will help you when you start your decluttering and resizing plan.*

Chapter Three

TOUGH LOVE ON TIDYING UP

*S*o, what is decluttering, and why does it matter?

de·clut·ter
/ˈdēklətər/

verb
*Remove unnecessary items from an untidy or overcrowded
place.*
"There's no better time to declutter your home."

In short, decluttering is getting rid of things that are not useful or meaningful, to create a tidy and harmonious space.

HERE IS A TEST:

- Do you spend a lot of time looking for everyday things?
- Do you know where important papers are, like passports, birth certificates or legal documents, and can you access them quickly in an emergency?

- Do you frequently replace items you can't find, only to find them later?
- Do you have rooms you can't go into because they are so full of stuff?
- Would you be mortified if anyone "dropped by" without calling first?
- Can you sit at the bar and dining table without having to bushwhack a path to a flat surface?
- Do you flinch when you open a cabinet or closet in case something falls out and hits you on the head?

If you answered yes to even one of these, a good declutter might be in order.

This is not a fun way to live: frustrated, always trying to find something, feeling like you just can't get it together. I am here to tough-love you, and tell you that you can, and you will!

The first important step you took was reading this book! That tells me you want to do this, and you are ready to change your mindset and lifestyle.

Consider that clutter has many negative statistics. Increased chances for falls or tripping are the most common, but too much stuff and clutter can also have health risks most people don't think about.

When there is a lot of clutter, cleaning isn't as thorough, giving mites and dust places to settle and increasing allergies and breathing problems. Bugs and rodents are also attracted to clutter because of lack of cleanliness and places to hide out. Both can be very damaging to property, and rodents carry a variety of dangerous diseases.

Clutter can impede your ability to get out of a home quickly in an emergency like a fire, and make fires easier to start, and spread more rapidly.

Clutter can create social isolation when people are embarrassed to have others over to their home. It becomes more of a hideout than a happy place to be.

Lastly, there is research that links obesity and weight gain to clutter. Too much stuff leads to inactivity, inability to work out or get exercise, and a sedentary lifestyle that encourages weight gain. Are these things you want MORE of in your life? The statistics on clutter are a bit overwhelming:

Many Americans who have a garage use it as a catchall. GarageLiving.com says that 25% of Americans with a garage never park a car in it, 50% of folks with a garage say it is the most disorganized space in their home and, when surveyed, they said "removing junk" was the top answer on how they could enjoy the space more.[1]

80% of items people keep are NEVER used according to PickupPlease.org, and they also found that people with extremely cluttered homes are 77% more likely to be overweight.[2]

Mother.ly found that women's stress levels are directly proportional to the amount of stuff in their homes, and that people are more productive, less irritable and less distracted in a clutter-free environment.[3]

I was really stunned by a study from ApartmentTherapy.com that shows Americans spend $2.7 Billion each year replacing things they cannot find! And 2.5 days a year looking for those same lost things![4]

Sadly, 54% of Americans are overwhelmed by the amount of clutter they have, and 78% have no idea what to do with it according to PRNewsWire.com.[5] The same research concluded that **getting rid of clutter eliminates 40% of the housework in an average home!**[6]

One final note on decluttering: as you complete areas and spaces, **make time to celebrate your wins!** Get a treat at Starbucks, have something special door dashed to your home, go have happy hour with a friend. Do SOMETHING to celebrate your success. I am bad at this, but I am getting better!

CHAPTER ACTION STEPS:

1. *Is clutter keeping you from fully living your life (be brutally honest about this, only you will see this answer)?*
2. *What would a decluttered home offer you?*
3. *Are you willing to make the effort to do some hard work to improve your life on so many levels by simply decluttering?*

Chapter Four

ISN'T RESIZING FOR OLD PEOPLE?

Resize
verb
re·size ()rē-ˈsīz
resized; resizing
transitive verb
: to make (something) a different size
took her ring to be resized
spent the morning resizing *images for the website*
gerund or present participle: **downsizing**
Make (something) smaller.
"I downsized the rear wheel to 26 inches."

ome ownership is widely considered the American dream.
Somewhere along the line, it was just a home, it wasn't a
home that was bigger and better than our friends', coworkers', or relatives'. It became about status, or in my line of work what we call a
"monument to your earning power."

Downsizing, right sizing, resizing: all terms that mean to "make
smaller." But resizing can also be living without excess, living more
simply and at a lower cost, with less energy spent on upkeep, mainte-

nance, housekeeping and managing things. I see it as making things more efficient on every level.

It also has a significant economic impact that has even more meaning as our country enters a new recession. Many families are priced out of home ownership, and many renting are being forced to look for smaller properties, or worse, face housing insecurity. Each day, I see more and more families living in their cars, or RV's. Housing prices have shot up exponentially, while incomes have barely kept up with the cost of living.

For some, smaller living is a preemptive strike to insulate their expenses and maintain housing, and for others, it's a choice to offset the higher cost of living and still allow them some financial freedom.

So, who is resizing for, and why am I so excited about it?

Resizing is for everyone, and it is a mindset. There's no minimum or maximum square footage. There are no special rules. It really applies to each person and family individually. But resizing is about living the best quality of life in a wonderful space. It's not about going without. It's certainly not minimalism. I often refer to it as "right-sizing." Picking and choosing the best of what you have, to enjoy fully in the space that works well for you!

Resizing is not about deprivation. For years, we lived in a large home and in the early 2000s, we sold a 4000 square foot home and "resized" to 3400 square feet. We currently live in 1131 square feet (if you had told me that 10 years ago, I would have been sure you had lost your mind!) and it's the best decision we've ever made. Period. It also doesn't mean going without. There is no rule about resizing, just some guidelines to help you choose the space you need. You can still have a guest room, office or hobby space, large kitchen, whatever you need and want.

So, what's in it for you to resize? It can be for people like us, who realized, once our daughter went off to college, that we didn't need all that house anymore. It can be for smaller families that either don't want the expense of a larger home or, more likely, can't afford the home that they'd ideally really like when weighing up economic times, cost of living, and the shortage of affordable housing.

Resizing makes a lot of sense, financially. Living in a smaller home generally creates lower living expenses. It gives you the opportunity to value experiences over things. It can be a catalyst to no mortgage or a lower mortgage. And it can give you a simpler, better quality of life. Not just for old people; for everyone.

You hear about couples whose kids have left home who are thinking about selling the big house and traveling. Or folks who are getting older who don't want to manage such a large home. But resizing isn't limited to an age group. Resizing is really about managing your stuff and your space. You can declutter possessions to create more space, or you can resize your stuff and your house to create simpler living.

When I began my resizing process, it was at the tail end of a very difficult recession. The recession of 2008 changed my outlook toward the future. And as I write this book, in the fall of 2022, we're right back there, heading into another recession, with many unknowns around the corner.

The great advantage of resizing, for me, is the ability to pick and choose the way I want to live, instead of waiting until I have no choice. Maybe when I'm older, I will have to move into an even smaller home, or an assisted living situation or some other smaller living situation than I'm used to. If and when that time comes, I'll be prepared.

When we're forced to do anything, it's usually a bitter pill. Almost everyone I've worked with who has had a major life transition requiring resizing did so not because they decided it was time, but because it was forced on them by health, finances, or family. It was a very tough, emotional journey for them, in most cases because of major life changes that caused or forced the move. And so many of these people did not want to move, let alone let go of their things. This wasn't an exciting proposition for them. They faced it with dread, and they felt like their belongings and their lives were being stripped down in front of them.

Having witnessed it several times, that's not a point I ever want to get to. And I also want to live a richer, fuller life and not be spending my time, energy, and resources shuffling through clutter, paying for maintenance that I don't need, paying high property taxes and people to take care of things that I can't or don't have time to, and I can use those funds in other ways.

Housing costs continue to spiral, whether rents or sales prices, driving many to the brink of housing insecurity. The economy is always going to be in a situation where housing prices are continually going up. When they're not, it's usually in a difficult and challenging recession. Cost of Living always increases, and as it does, I see so many struggling not only to find a home of their dreams, but in many cases lately, justifying the home they can afford. Choosing to live smaller, while still challenging for some, can be an offset to the very high cost of living.

I've noticed a large movement of families going to live in RVs full time, homeschooling their kids while traveling around the country. What an amazing way to raise your kids! Now that so many people can work from anywhere, it's truly possible. The options are limitless. And so, I just ask you to open your mind to the many possibilities that could come your way as a benefit of resizing your belongings and home.

Americans live with so much clutter. Amazon delivers stuff to your house every day. Admit it! I'll raise my hand, too. But I look carefully at those new arrivals and decide which ones are important to me, where they will live, and what I need and want to keep over just keeping everything because I ordered it.

Everything has a time and season and anything that can be replaced easily, I don't have a lot of hesitation in getting rid of. It's often the sentimental items that trip people up. But I have a plan.

The pushback will start for many of you almost immediately. "Well, I don't want my kids to have to share a bedroom," "I'm not ready to part with my stuff." Since you picked up this book, you clearly have a desire to live more simply on some level. So read on with an open mind. No timeline, just thinking about the possibilities.

Resizing is not just going to become more popular for the simplicity it offers, but because of the costs. More people are already looking to resize to prevent cash flow issues or overspending. Many cities, towns, and counties don't allow people to live in a tiny home or RV on their own land (nope, I am not joking, it is illegal in many counties in my state). So how do we help people live more economically when times are so challenging and costly? Smaller homes, home shares, and rentable apartments where allowed by code will all increase in popularity.

My message to you is this: only you can decide whether a resized home is for you. But decluttering is a commitment to manage your things before they manage you. It's a decision that requires continual action.

CHAPTER ACTION STEPS:

1. *How could resizing impact your life in a positive way? More time, money, energy?*
2. *How would you spend your time, energy and money if you had MORE of it?*
3. *What sorts of features and spaces would you need in a resized home for it to feel fully functional?*

Chapter Five

AMERICA, LAND OF THE STORAGE UNITS

*J*ust driving around, have you ever noticed how many storage units there are in your town? There's one on almost every corner where I live, and they're full of stuff, maybe even your stuff. And for a few years they were full of my stuff. Not anymore. I'm not saying I don't have a box or two on a shelf. I do. But I know exactly what is in them, and why I am keeping them in boxes, not in a storage unit.

Did you know that US Self Storage Industry statistics prove that 9.4% of all US households rent a storage unit?[1] Or that 67% of self-storage renters live in a home with a garage, and 33% also have a basement? Or that 52% rent storage space for a year or more at an average monthly cost of close to $100 a month?[2]

When my husband's grandfather passed away, his grandmother was able to live in their home for many years. But as her health failed, we needed to move her to a smaller apartment. An incredible cook and noted local dinner party hostess, she had a lot of possessions to process. Because she wasn't quite ready to part with all of her things, we rented a storage unit while we tirelessly sorted through items with her, and while she thought she was doing a great job resizing, we still had a large storage unit full of goods that we couldn't fit into her new one-bedroom apartment. These items stayed in storage for years.

Let's just say that, at $100 a month, it may have cost her close to $5,000 over the years that it was stored. My husband's grandparents had been successful business owners and enjoyed a very comfortable retirement, but because of increased costs, eventually her money got tight, and she had to let go of the storage unit and all the things in it. I remember feeling so sad that she had spent all that money to save those things that ultimately ended up being sold at a garage sale. Yes, a few small treasures were passed on, but for the most part, she spent $5,000 for the peace of mind of knowing that her things were a few miles away and she could have a family member retrieve them at any time. She often visited her storage unit with relatives. Her possessions were THAT important to her. I have often wondered if, after her money was gone, she would have chosen to use that money in a different way?

There are many benefits to decluttering and resizing. I hope these are obvious by now, but let's recap:

- Having a more organized, less cluttered home. No matter the size. Having a place for things, knowing exactly what you have, and finding them easily. Less unnecessary replacing of existing items and much less time searching for those items.
- No more embarrassment when someone just stops by and knocks on the door wanting to come in. Feeling ready to entertain at a moment's notice.
- Lower cost of living. Less money paid for utilities, taxes, maintenance and upkeep, insurance, repairs, possessions. You get to keep more of your money when you live smaller.
- The ability to entertain more, and more comfortably. Not a draw for some, but for many it's an ideal!
- Saving the money you've been spending on storage for something more meaningful. Maybe to upgrade your home? Perhaps you'd like hardwood floors or new carpet. Remodel

your kitchen or bathroom. Buy a nice piece of art. Make your home a more personal reflection of the people who live there. Or maybe a month-long trip to Europe? More experiences, trips to the zoo as a family because you have more money and time you're no longer spending to maintain a huge home and its contents.

Turn that space you can't walk into because it's crammed with stuff into something functional and beautiful. Maybe a guest room so you could have company over? Or perhaps you have a big enough home that you could supplement your income by creating a rental space to list on Airbnb, or rent to a roommate? I am a firm believer that physical clutter is mental and emotional clutter. When I, or others declutter, it's a change in energy, and it works! Resizing allows for new experiences; less stuff and less space make this all possible. There are other great reasons to declutter and resize. Some people have very large homes that they're not using, but all the rooms are full. Even if you aren't going to resize your home, there are still significant benefits to resizing your stuff.

CHAPTER ACTION STEPS:

1. *What are the main problem areas in your home that need decluttering?*
2. *How much money annually are you spending on storage? Include the cost of rent, sheds, temporary heat, and storage containers/bins, you have purchased.*
3. *What would you do MORE of if your home was decluttered or you were able to resize? Entertain? Travel? Save for retirement? Something else?*

Chapter Six

MINDSET AND OVERCOMING ROADBLOCKS TO SUCCESS

There are many common themes or blocks that come up, and I have laid them out in **bold**.

I think the first really important step in any decluttering process is **understanding your organizational style.** That is, if you want the habits to stick.

There's an amazing book by Cassandra Aarssen, called The Clutter Connection. You can visit her website at www.clutterbug.me. She offers a free, easy quiz to tell you what your organizational style is and what type of clutterbug you are.

My own family all took this test in the not-too-distant past, and I was really surprised at the results. In my house, we have three members in our family and three different types of clutterbugs.

I am Cricket, a classic organizer. I crave visual simplicity, and detailed organizing systems. I don't want or have to see my stuff to know it is there. I like things put away in cabinets or drawers, not out all over the counters and other surfaces.

My husband is a Bee. He likes visual abundance, seeing his things, and likes detailed organization systems. He likes to keep things out that he is working on until he is done. He has some pills he takes right before bed, so each night he sets them in a small dish after dinner to remind himself to take them before going to sleep.

Our daughter is a Butterfly. She craves visual abundance and super simple organizing systems. For her "out of sight" means completely out of mind. She needs to leave her vitamins out on the counter to remember to take them.

Once I understood this as the main organizer in our home, it made things SO much easier to manage. When I understood the needs of each person, I was able to make some tweaks to our household system that worked well for all of us, and helped keep us on track.

It also helped me help my family members stay organized. For example, my husband struggles with organization in his workshop, which he shares with our employees. Once I understood his organizational style, I was able to help him think of better ways to manage his shop items.

The next step is **mindset**. You really must spend some time thinking about this process, and I will include some tips on letting go in this chapter from a psychotherapist friend.

Your headspace is everything. If someone else wants you to declutter and resize, it will never happen. If you want someone else to declutter and resize and they are not interested, you're going to be pushing a boulder up the hill.

Hard conversations are often needed. If you have a partner, spouse or other family members, a family meeting , or maybe a few, might be necessary to talk about the group goal and how you're going to get there and what everybody's part will be. It's important that everybody is on board. If you're having to resize or declutter because of life circumstances, that can be extra hard. Counseling can be helpful. Talking it out with a trusted friend can be beneficial. But you also must really spend some time deciding what you want and how you're going to get there. Period.

Are you going to resist change and be stubborn? Are you going to be difficult? Are you going to be cooperative? But also, are you going to stand your ground and be participatory?

It's never fun to help someone resize who doesn't want to. Everything becomes stressful and emotional. The person downsizing feels attacked and uncared for. If you can get in the right headspace in advance, you'll be miles ahead.

There are lots of emotional aspects of decluttering and resizing. I hear a lot of people say they never want to leave their home because they had so many memories there, and I love that. But I also know that **memories are portable**. They don't belong to any one place. Yes, the memory happened at that home or that space. But that memory goes with you; it doesn't go away when you leave. The memory does not fade when the object is gone.

When I was a child, I used to watch my grandpa shave when I visited. He would wet his shaving brush, lather up the soap in what looked to me like a coffee mug, brush that foamy mess all over his face, and shave it off. When he was done, he would turn the crank handle on his old-school metal razor to open the top, and remove the straight razor blade. Then he would lather up my face and help me "shave" too. When he passed, my grandma offered the mug to me, and I did not take it. For years, I regretted that, but finally realized the memory is still just as strong without the physical reminder of the mug.

Are there physical aspects in the house that you don't want to part with? For example, a wall where you measured all your children or grandchildren? There are ways to preserve that. But the emotional aspect encompasses so many things. Very few of these decisions are meant to be life or death. You just want to be honest about the importance of keeping something.

I asked Kirsten Friedman, Licensed Mental Health Counselor and truly awesome human being, (Certified Psychodramatist, TEP, Certified Therapist - Internal Family Systems) to help you with an exercise in mindset and letting go. Let's dive in!

We can feel a lot of internal resistance when we consider letting go of our stuff. Maybe there's a part that's scared to get rid of things, or that feels sad at the thought of abandoning certain items, or that craves the comfort of being surrounded by the tangible feeling of home and security. Maybe there are parts that freeze us in our tracks when we try to get rid of stuff and distract us with online shopping, or a trip to Trader Joe's frozen treats section. Maybe there are parts that feel frustrated and angry that we can't let go, or even ashamed that we can't seem to clear our space. And then we don't even want to think about any of it.

The Internal Family Systems (IFS) model of looking at our own minds might be helpful in untangling the snarl of feelings and thoughts that come up when we get serious about letting go of our stuff. IFS says that we are all made up of parts. We each have a Self that is calm, clear, confident and courageous (among other qualities), that we have had since birth and that cannot be destroyed. And we each have many other parts that we have had to "grow" to deal with what life has dealt us.

These other parts have their own skills and attributes. We experience some as useful (like that part that knows how to organize a mess, or to break the ice in a new relationship). Some parts may feel more problematic: the part that absolutely snaps when we are cut off in traffic, the part that others tell us is "bossy," the part that cannot help but reach for a donut when we feel a certain way (lonely, or anxious, or sad, maybe).

The message of IFS is: "All parts are good. Each of them is trying to help us in its own way."

IFS divides parts into three groups: managers, firefighters and exiles. The managers are proactive protectors. They are out in front of things organizing, or relating to people, or taking care of life to make sure we are taken care of. The firefighters are reactive protectors. Like emergency responders, they swoop in when life gets past our managers and feels (to the firefighters) like we have to be rescued from whatever just happened (even if it's just an icky feeling, or a disturbing thought). These firefighters, which can include things like shopping, or scrolling, or eating, or alcohol, or marijuana or other drugs, essentially hijack the system and take us momentarily to a "safe" space. But, after their heroic deed, our system is often flooded with shame and remorse, which puts us a little closer to "needing them" again.

The last parts, the "exiles," are the parts of us tucked deep away in our psyches that hold the experiences or feelings that were just too awful to deal with when they happened. The experiences may have been terrible by any definition—the death of a parent when we were children, the death of a beloved childhood pet, abandonment by friends or loved ones, any kind of physical, emotional or sexual abuse, etc. Or, the experiences may have been less dramatic, but made intolerable to our insides because there was no one around to help us navigate them—a crushing disappointment at school or in a competition, being unpopular at school, missing out on something we yearned for. The protector parts, firefighters and managers, valiantly work hard to prevent these exiles from being hurt again. They do this either by trying to control what happens to us in advance (the managers), or by hijacking the situation and taking everyone to what feels like momentary safety (the firefighters).

IFS says we all have these parts. Every single human being.

What does this have to do with getting rid of stuff? Here is an exercise that uses IFS to help us let go of things we no longer need.

IFS EXERCISE FOR LETTING GO

In a quiet, calm moment, take out a piece of paper and, in the middle of it, write something like: "I would like to/need to get rid of some things/clutter." Use your own words so it's meaningful to you.

Then, wait for a feeling to come up.

When one comes up, say "anxiety," for example, place it somewhere on the page, where it feels like it belongs. You can draw it, or write it. You can use color. You can make it as far away or as close to what you originally wrote as it feels like it should be. Then wait for the next thing to come up. Maybe it's "sadness." Maybe "overwhelm." Try to welcome the feeling and thank it for showing up. Put it too on the piece of paper, in any place or way that feels right. Then wait for the next one.

If a firefighter shows up, like "forget this exercise, just go get a cookie," write *that* down, too.

Keep doing this process until it feels like all your feelings are out on the page.

This is like a map of your feelings around clearing space. See what it feels like to look at all of them. Remember, as you look at them, that they are ALL trying to help you, and that none of them are bad, just worried about the young exiles they are protecting.

If you want to declutter your space, you will have to make friends with all the parts on your map. You can do this from Self-energy, that place in you where you feel calm, courageous, confident, clear, compassionate, connected, curious, and creative. From this place, or as much of it as you can muster, let each part know you are going to take care of them and keep them safe. Get to know them a little. Find out what makes them do their job for you. If they are sad, what are they sad about? If anxious, what are they afraid will happen? If they get overwhelmed, what are they afraid will paralyze them? Let them know you're not going to make them go away; you are going to help them be ok with what you need to do.

Then, use this newfound friendship to actually take care of them. Maybe you have a box of stuff to go to Goodwill. Your anxious part won't let you take it out of the trunk, and you've been driving around with it for months. Pull up your Self-energy, and ask the part that is afraid what will happen if you take it out and hand it to the worker at Goodwill? Listen to the part. Ask it what it needs from *you* to allow it to let go. Maybe it needs to know that you will still be safe and ok without that particular box. Maybe it needs to know that dropping off that box won't lead to you getting rid of everything you own. Work with it.

Remember it's just a part of you, and that it means well. Don't force it. Our parts want to move toward health and harmony. If they feel safe and welcome by you, they will shift.

If you'd like more information about IFS, you can go to their website, ifs-institute.com/. There is also an easy-to-read book explaining the model: No Bad Parts: Healing Trauma and Restoring Wholeness with the Internal Family Systems Model by Richard Schwartz, Ph.D.

If, in trying this practice, you discover that the root of some of these parts feels too difficult/scary for you to handle on your own, think about getting some coaching or therapy. If you like the IFS model, there is a directory of IFS therapists on the website above. Many therapists work online, so you are not restricted to finding someone local. If the IFS model doesn't really click with you, do consider getting some help from a coach or therapist, maybe someone who specializes in helping folks let go. The main thing to know is that you don't have to suffer this alone.

There are many modalities, IFS being only one. If this model doesn't work well for you, there are many techniques on mindset and letting go available in book form, on the internet, and even through counseling or therapy. Whatever works best for you!

There are many **emotional aspects** that play into decluttering and resizing.

Control issues tend to pop up when a person is decluttering because they waited to the point where it is "do or die." This is commonly older parents or relatives, people with health issues, maybe financial issues, people who *must* resize. And when people lose control over where they're living and what's happening, they tend to grasp other things and that control can then be transferred to their belongings. And so, it becomes even harder for them to part with many of these things.

Poverty or lack of funds is another emotional trigger. Many people who haven't had much money, or worked really hard to get the things, are afraid of giving them up because they worry they'll never be able to replace them.

Fear of change can make people grasp a bit more tightly, and often comes out in the form of "Well, I'm not sure what I'll need in my new place," so they want to take it all with them. Are you going to regret decluttering and getting rid of things? Are you going to wish you hadn't given away your grandmother's clock? Or your grandfather's pocket watch? Are those things going to come back and haunt you? That's a big one for people. They worry that they're going to make a decision they will regret.

Lack of a simple organization structure can also impact people's ability to let go of things. If you don't know what you really have, how do you know what you really need and what you can let go of? Many people avoid decluttering because they lack organizational structure.

Attachment or transition can be challenging. Attachment to items can come up if they belonged to a person who is deceased. It's all they have left of their loved one. There are ways to keep those things as part of your decor or even your daily life so that they're useful and meaningful. Not stuffed in the back of a cabinet or closet. Look at items with fresh eyes. How can I incorporate this into my daily life? Because it is special, try making it part of daily life instead of just having it somewhere in your house where you can't even see it. The hardest part for many people is the emotional component and doing the work ahead of time to really think about what's important.

Depression Era Folks are notorious for their difficulty in parting with possessions. My grandma Fran was a child during the depression, but she recalled it vividly. My Grandpa ate his toast black and burned because as a child in the depression living at a logging camp, the loggers got the "good" toast, and the children all ate the burned toast so as not to waste it. Grandpa lived to be 77 and told me that if the toaster wasn't smoking, the toast wouldn't be done. Fran saved margarine wrappers all year long. Imperial margarine, you know (if you are of a certain age), the one with the crown. She saved them because they were foil, and she used them at Thanksgiving and Christmas to wrap the baked potatoes in so that, when baking, the littlest bits of margarine left on the foil would not go to waste, but would soak into the potato skin. There is a wasteful mindset that depression era folks can't tolerate and will require a special level of making sure anything that is leaving is still going to be of use, and not become trash.

Lastly, **perfectionism**. There's a saying I love: "perfect is the enemy of done." Originally "The perfect is the enemy of the good," - Volatire. And I say that as an admitted perfectionist. I like things to be done the best they can. But I've realized in the last decade or so that it's more important to complete some tasks than to just talk about them and wait to do them until the time is perfect. This book is a great example. I've been talking about writing this book for years, decades actually, and finally writing and publishing it gives me a great sense of completing something I've been dreaming about for a long time. For some people, that's resizing and decluttering; they just don't know where to start and are waiting for the perfect time.

There's an old Facebook meme that I saw again the other day about how some grown children were helping their older parents or grandparents declutter. Here is it is, in case you've never seen it:

A friend posted this writing today and it struck me that someday EVERYONE will go through this discarding of "things" that are the memories of one's life. Sometimes it's our own and more often it's the life of someone we love.....

When my mom was cleaning out her house over 23 years ago to sell it, I wasn't very sympathetic over her attachments to things. I would go over on weekends to help her, and we would go through things, things for a yard sale, things to donate, things to throw away. I would usually get upset over how long it took her to decide. For instance, we were going through kitchen cabinets, and she spent 20 minutes looking at an iron kettle with a lid. Finally, I said, "Mom, at this rate it is going to take us another 2 years."

She told me that her mother used to make meals in that kettle and leave them at the doorsteps of neighbors during the depression. Mom would deliver them, and then they would reappear back to her with an apron, or a wood carving, something in return for the meal. I realized that everything that my mom was going through was really a reliving of her life.

If you are reading this and are under the age of 60, you won't get it. You haven't lived long enough. Most of you have not had to move your parents into a nursing home, or emptied their home. You haven't lived long enough to realize that the hours you spend picking out the right cabinets, or the perfect tile will not be what matters in the later years. It will be the handmade toothbrush holder, or a picture that you got on vacation.

So, if your parents are resizing, and moving to smaller places, or selling a home, give your mom and even your dad a break. Those things that you don't understand why they can't just pitch, and why you think you know what needs to be tossed or saved, give them a little time to make their decisions. They are saying goodbye to their past and realizing that they are getting ready for their end of life, while you are beginning your life.

As I have been going through things, it's amazing just how hard it is to get rid of objects. But life goes on, and you realize they are just things, but sometimes things comfort us. So, give your parents or grandparents a break. Listen to their stories, because in 40 years, when you are going through those boxes and the memories come back, it will be hard to get rid of those plastic champagne flutes that you and your late husband used at a New Year's party 40 years ago. You will think nothing of the tile or the light fixtures that were so important then.

As happy as they are for you, and as much as they love you, you just don't have a clue until it happens to you and then you will remember how you rushed them, and it will make you sad, especially if they are already gone and you can't say, "I'm sorry, I didn't get it."

— *ORIGINAL POST, MELISSA VAUGHAN*

In the story, the kids are rushing the parents, the kids get impatient, and the parents get upset and the whole situation gets tense. In the end, the story says you've rushed these people through their memories and their life and when they're gone, you'll be sorry that you did that. And you can't possibly understand if you are under the age of 60.

This story only represents one side. And a sad one, admittedly. No one wants to part with treasured belongings, or be forced to move, yet it happens to most older Americans at some point due to health care needs, finances, lack of family support and other reasons.

However, let's look at the flip side of this story. From my experience, which I admit is limited in a world view, many of the people I have worked with had been offered help by family earlier in the game, and either rejected it, or did it on a very limited basis. By the time the move WAS imminent, there was now this overwhelming timeline to get things sorted and the family member moved. The tension had already built up, and this can result in a disastrous "clean out" that leaves the family member feeling hurt and disrespected. That is where I have been many times, and it is equally painful.

Tough love time. I'm including this story so we can look at *both* sides and hopefully heed the warning. **What we are unwilling to control, in the end, will control us.** Be willing to look ahead and think about what might happen, and how *you* want to have it unfold. I firmly believe that we're all in charge of where we end up. Simple accountability. And if you aren't willing to do the work, declutter and resize now, someone will be assigned to help you do it. It sounds so harsh, but the truth sometimes is. That doesn't mean it isn't true.

Feeling forced is never easy, nor fun. It's much easier for you to manage your life and things now on your own terms.

The other thing to think about, especially if you're older, and you've got an accumulation of a lifetime, is being the person left with the mess. I encourage you to ask yourself this VERY difficult question: Do you really want to keep all the things and leave your house in chaos to your children or some other relative to clean up after you're gone? That's a huge physical and emotional burden for your kids or your family members. I say this from experience. That alone is enough to move most people to thinking *"I don't want to be that way. I'm going to manage myself."*

In general, there will be plenty of crap for our daughter to deal with when we are gone. I don't wish to burden her with a giant mess I could have dealt with. I am not advocating insensitivity, rushing people or being aggressive. I am hoping people understand their *roles* in this process. Do you own the stuff or does the stuff own you?

If there was a fire, and you had 5 minutes to pack, what would you take? Keep that, the rest can be replaced. Do the work and help yourself. There is a saying I believe in here, "God helps those who help themselves." It's a powerful truth. Drive the car yourself, or you will be driven. The choice is 100% up to you.

Yes, listen to their stories, help them make decisions, and help them to figure out how to take a piece of it with them, or the memory with them. An item does not always have to be used for its original intent to remain useful.

FAMILY CONSENSUS ABOUT DECLUTTERING

What is the family situation? Is everyone living in the house on board? Or will they be dragged along kicking and screaming?

I have seen a husband-and-wife bicker about the other's crap and refuse to part with theirs unless the spouse parts with some too. Seriously, is that working for you?

How can you come together, how can you work towards agreement? Do you each have a space and once it's full, hard choices need to be made? This is where letting go really can be helpful. Why is it you feel the need to keep certain things? Don't shake your head and say you don't know, search for the *why*...it's there, and it might be a little challenging to admit, but unearth that reason and see if it is something you truly require, or if you can part with some or all of it.

You will need to get everyone on board for a timeline. When do you want it to be done? Who will help, what will you do with the stuff that's leaving, what supplies do you need, how will you decide what stays and goes (in the next chapter, I will spill the beans on all that). Some families will benefit from counseling, coaching, therapy or a professional to help them through this process.

Every time I did a major move with a family member or friend's family member, I would come home and look at my own stuff with new eyes. And ultimately, I chose a giant resize for myself.   Sure, we still have plenty of stuff. And no estate is ever going to be a piece of cake to settle. There are always going to be belongings. But think about what you're really leaving behind for your kids. Is that what you want to do? That's a very important takeaway.

I was raised in a family that got rid of things they didn't need. My mom made regular trips to Goodwill. She didn't over-buy. But when she was done with something or it was no longer needed, she would give it away to a charity to sell.

My husband was raised in a family that once you owned something, you just kept it, because you paid for it. That makes a lot of sense. However, if you've had an electric wok sitting up in the kitchen cabinet above your refrigerator for 25 years, and it's so covered in dust that you'd have to scrub it within an inch of its life to use it? I'm going to go out on a limb and say it's probably something you don't need. Yes, you paid for it. Yes, it has value. But why not put it into the hands of someone else who could benefit from it?

I always suggest that people pick a small space to get started. Nothing crazy. A medicine cabinet. A bathroom drawer. The junk drawer. Well, let's not start there. That might be a little overwhelming. The silverware drawer.

I love task timers, the kind you can just flip and do a task at a time for a preset duration. I have one that I use almost every day in increments of five to 60 minutes. You flip it to the minutes you want, and you go like hell. When the timer goes off, you're usually very surprised at what you could accomplish in a short amount of time. 5, 10, 15 minutes. And often people say, "Well, that wasn't so bad. I could do five more minutes, or I could do 15 more minutes."

This is how you start.

I want you to always consider what's easily replaceable. When you're going through items, have a threshold in mind: if this is replaceable for less than $20 (or whatever you feel is reasonable), that is your cut-off guideline. There'll be a little gray area. You know that extra frying pan might come in handy. Well, it might. But if your pots and pans are overflowing, maybe it's time for the rattiest pan to go. And when you need a new pan, you can pick one up from any variety of sources, from free to full retail.

CHAPTER ACTION STEPS:

1. *Is your mindset ready for this process, and have you gone through the mindset exercise?*
2. *Where in the process do you think you will have the most trouble, and how do you plan to overcome that?*
3. *If there are other household members, who might be the most resistant to this process and how can you work with them to create change?*

Chapter Seven

YOUR BLUEPRINT FOR SUCCESS

*Y*ou're ready to start the big declutter. The sort and purge.

Planning is key. I believe any successful project or outcome starts with planning. As a homebuilder, I plan everything on paper before I ever stick a shovel in the ground. A successful plan can be easily implemented, whereas no plan gives you poor results. It's important to make time to plan this out. And your plan should take your particular needs into consideration.

What do you need to prepare for? Think about your goal: are you just decluttering room by room? Cleaning out a separate building like a barn or shop, maybe a garage?

Let's lay out the steps to your plan for the decluttering process!

MAKE AGREEMENTS

Make sure everyone in your home is on the same page. This can honestly be the biggest sticking point for many.

If you are single, you only need your own agreement...easy! If you are married or have a partner...totally different story. When talking with some of my friends about the differences in how they declutter vs their spouse/partner...oh my, night and day! And on a fairly regular basis, each partner or spouse has a totally different mindset.

Some folks are the "tit for tat" types. *"If I get rid of this, you need to get rid of that."* A heart to heart may be in order. Or one person may not want to play along at all. You can still proceed, but you will have to use caution.

When we did our major resize, I ran some items by my husband that were things in his domain. I don't cook, but I am a great dish-washer, grocery shopper and kitchen cleaner. So when pans came out of cupboards we had not seen in years, I asked for his input. There were some things we agreed to keep and, if we had not used them in a year, we would get rid of them.

Some couples have to divide space. For example, we do have a large shop for our business. Some of the stuff my husband doesn't want to part with goes to the shop. He has the room, and that is where it lives. So, worst case, you can assign space to each partner, with an agreement about what will happen when that space is at capacity.

For the record, my husband was not an active participant in the declutter. But I did run things by him at the end of each declutter day to get his take, so he didn't feel like I was getting rid of things without his consent. That can create an entirely new problem. This arrange-ment worked well for us. Find the method that works for you! But do it up-front and have some ground rules, or it will not be successful.

TIME-BOX IT

Especially if you are decluttering with the idea of having a big garage/estate sale, set the date for the sale or when you wish the decluttering to be completed by. A project with a deadline is much more likely to reach completion than one without.

CLARIFY YOUR GOALS

Don't just think about them, actually write out a list of goals. What are you decluttering (space wise), when will you work on it, with whom, how will things leaving be handled, and what date will you be complete? Post this where it can be easily seen every day! Are there specific days or times you will work on this? Add that to the calendar, along with who will be helping if you have a helper. Add these goals to the shared family calendar so you get reminders or times when you have planned to do some decluttering.

GATHER YOUR SUPPLIES

A few large plastic bins with lids that can be stacked up full or empty are very helpful for sorting. I recommend 6 very large bins/tubs. Large trash bags tend to be the easiest to use for donations, but you can also use boxes picked up from local stores, if those are more manageable. Also, a spiral notebook for noting anything you might store in boxes.

HAVE AN EXIT STRATEGY

Plan on HOW you will deal with the stuff that is leaving. If items are being gifted or donated, they need to leave the house the day you declutter them. This keeps them from mysteriously going back to their original spot, second-guessing, and additional clutter of bags or boxes clogging up halls and entryways. Load them in the car and *get rid of them*. Or hire someone to drop them off for you.

One way people get tripped up is by wanting to gift items to specific friends, family or nonprofits. This keeps the items in the house and in the way. Make a rule about these items. Friends or family pickup within 2 days, or they are delivered to them. Just have a clear rule that is reasonable about this, or you will create a sticking point here very quickly. I suggest an unattached party to be your helper and possibly delivery person. Set aside a small area for these items to be held in but keep the time limit short to keep momentum going.

IDENTIFY YOUR HELPERS

Though household members really ought to be your front-line helpers, that is not always the case. Sometimes they're unable, or simply unwilling, to participate in the process. Do you have friends, church, or civic group friends? Can you hire an organizer, or local person to help sort, or to drop off to donation centers or friends you are gifting to? Do you need to hire an estate salesperson or auctioneer (for some homes, this is needed and well worth the cost)?

GET AN ACCOUNTABILITY PARTNER

You know, someone you tell your goals to, and they help you stick with it. This is best if they are not also part of the declutter. An unattached party. Tell them your plans and dates and check in with them often. Reward yourself for specific milestones.

JUST DO IT!

Grab a task timer and just start, going room by room or space by space. The task timer is not to rush you. It is to help you set up motivated microbursts of work.

If you think you can't start in a room because you only have 15 minutes, just start and work for 15 minutes; you will often find you can keep going. Keep track of where you left off with a sticky note.

Touch *everything*. No skipping stuff for later.

Open every box, even if it's labeled. When my grandma left her large house of almost 50 years, there was a lot of stuff there. The clean-up effort was led by two of her three grown daughters, and not the most sentimental ones, so that was already not in her favor. My grandpa had passed years before, so it was just my grandma, my mom and an aunt making the calls.

As time wore on, the daughters got more impatient. One had flown up from California to help and time was running out on her stay. It came down to a lot of stuff that appeared to be trash just getting tossed in the dumpster without much of an inspection.

Years later, I asked why my grandpa's ashes were not in the headstone at his grave; the vault was empty. My grandma piped up that his ashes were in a box, but she wasn't sure where. A look came over my mom's face that wasn't good, as she turned to her own mother and asked what kind of box? Grandma described a kelly green shoe box, it had been in her bedroom closet on a shelf, but she did not know where it ended up.

I wasn't sure if my mom was going to cry or laugh next, but she laughed and told us that she knew exactly where Grandpa's ashes were. She and my aunt had lost a bit of patience at the end and the green shoebox looked like junk, so they tossed it into the dump trailer without a second thought. So, my grandpa's ashes were very unintentionally spread at the local dump. This was comical and ironic, because he used to take those same two girls to the dump when they were little to shoot at the rats with BB guns.

For some families, this would not be funny; it would be devastating, but for my warped gang, we laugh often about Grandpa's final resting place and how perfect it is for him. The moral of the story: if the box says hand mixer, or shoes, open it up and make sure of what is inside!

I have helped people who were leaving a home of 40 plus years. They were just taking the things they wanted to go with them, so we could easily go room by room and pull the things they wanted, leaving the rest behind for an estate sale or auctioneer (trust me, this is not "easy"). You must look at and touch things to decide what you are keeping.

If there has been a recent death, perhaps of a spouse, then I suggest something called "memorabilia tubs." In one case, we bought large purple bins with lids, into which were placed the belongings of a husband who had passed. No one was ready to process those items just yet, but we knew we did not want to simply toss or donate all of them. I don't advocate filling these to store for years; at some point you will need to process them. But if a death was recent and still too hard to deal with in the middle of a declutter and resize, it is OK to postpone some decisions for later to avoid overwhelm that could stop progress.

DON'T FORGET CLOTHES

I know people who have every closet in their home filled with clothes, *every one of them*, and there might only be 2 people living there. They keep every item of clothing they ever bought whether it fits or not.

CreditDonkey.com states the average family spends $1800 a year on clothing, and 32% of women have more than 25 pairs of shoes (so guilty, boots don't count as shoes though, right?)[1] and throw out 81 pounds of clothing per year![2]

Keeping unworn items drives me nuts, and here is why. Have you ever walked into a huge closet full of clothes and thought "I have nothing to wear." Yep, because you are keeping all the "too small" clothes "in case" you lose weight. Or you're hanging onto the too-big clothes from before you lost weight, just in case you gain a few pounds. I call this "fat insurance."

Stuff that itches, scratches, was expensive, someone gave it to you, pinches, the zipper is broken. Fill in the blanks. Fix it with a seamstress or get rid of it. Keep the clothes that you actually *wear*. That *fit*. Sure, toss a few oddballs on the storage rack or the back of a closet. The rest needs to go.

I was recently a house guest at a friend's. When I arrived, they showed me to the guest room. But there was no room in the guest room for my clothes. The room was smaller and full of a queen bed and large dresser, which was all it could accommodate. The closet was packed to the gills, as was the dresser. The closet door would not even slide open more than 2 inches. They told me to go ahead and put my suitcase in the office next door to the guest room, and I could use that room for my clothes. While I was very grateful for their hospitality, I was running back and forth in the hall in my PJ's trying to find all my things.

I recently completed a guest room in my small home. I had a queen Murphy bed installed. The room is small and when the bed is down, there is not a ton of space, but enough. I made sure that the closet has *dedicated* space for a guest's hanging items, hangers for them to use, a shelf for folded items, and a spot for their suitcase.

SORT TO BINS

In each room or space, sort to the bins. I generally label them Guilt, Give, Get, and Go (more on that in the next chapter), and boxes for anything you know will go to storage or be moved soon and you can live without. Any boxes for storage or moving need to be managed and have an area to stage them.

Manage these bins at the end of each sort. Pack the boxes, stage them, put the items to give away in your car and drop off , deliver, or schedule a pick-up in a short timeframe.

Be ruthless! Things are replaceable. Memories can be transported. Let me say it again for the people in the back!!! Look carefully at any furniture you have that can do double duty. Storage ottomans, dressers or chests that offer good storage and look nice can be a good sideboard or accent piece. Coffee tables that have space for baskets underneath can corral kid or dog toys, books, throw blankets and more.

Have an open mind about the things you own. I was recently visiting a friend who wanted better organization in an area of her house, and I gave her some suggestions. She looked at me a little puzzled and said, "but then I would have to buy a new piece of furniture when I already have this."

I must admit, I was a little dumbfounded. If your shoes don't fit, do you still wear them and just suffer from hurting feet? If your clothes are too tight, or the fabric is itchy, do you just make do? I understand the desire to not be frivolous. But for so many people, part of enjoying your home is enjoying the things and spaces in it! The beauty of it. How it makes you feel.

You can sell the old piece to help offset the cost of the newer item. You can buy something online that has been "previously loved," also known as "used"; you can make something. Get creative and don't limit yourself to what you have.

When we resized, I brought one piece of furniture with me. *One.* I bought all new, and while some may think that is a luxury (and I agree, it is), it is not impossible. There are many ways to do it from very reasonably to full retail. Take your pick. We also sold a lot of our belongings which funded most of my new furniture purchases. My new home is a very different scale in room size than my old home. Also, a very different architectural style, so I took the opportunity to furnish it the way that worked for the space and our needs, and it was a great choice for us.

Do you ever watch HGTV and listen to people looking at homes who say things like "I don't like the paint color," or "our couch would never fit in there." Folks, we can *change* things. It's not hard. A couch was not designed to last your entire life, and neither was the paint. Mix it up, have some fun, try something new.

If you plan to resize and move, add these steps:

You still need to follow the steps to declutter, but here are some added tips for those that will be making a move.

EMPTY THE SPACE COMPLETELY

When I sort a space, my goal is to *empty* the space and put back *only* what's staying.

Let's use closets as an example. My first step would be to empty it space by space. First any shelves, then any hanging items. You can do this one by one, or empty the whole mess onto the bed (that can be a bit overwhelming for some, so I often go section by section). Touch and process everything. If you're keeping it, it goes back. If it's leaving, it either gets packed for the move, or if in use, stays in place until the move is very close.

If you're keeping it and it needs cleaning, fixing, repairing, then create that task so it can be done. Put it in the car to go to the seamstress, place it in the laundry area if it needs stain treatment or washing - you get the idea. Don't put back anything that is NOT going to stay with you permanently. This becomes an easy go-to mechanism for dealing with challenging items and can become an easy avoidance technique.

MAKE IT REAL

Set a date for a garage or estate sale if you will be having one.

What is the move date, or what is the date you'll be listing your home? Working backwards from that date will help you to ensure that you're ready at the proper time.

PLAN FOR YOUR NEEDS

If you're moving, you may have some things to pack up. You're going to have some things to get rid of. So, what are you going to do for preparation there?

- Do you need to plan a garage sale?
- Do you need to plan for help packing?
- Do you need to look for a new home?
- Or do you need to speak to remodelers?

GATHER YOUR SUPPLIES

Moving boxes, packing tape, paper for wrapping, masking or painters' tape, larger blank labels, sharpies or markers, scissors and a spiral bound notebook will be helpful for tracking items packed for the move.

ESTABLISH A MOVING BOX STORAGE AREA

For items going into moving boxes, I label two sides of each box where they meet at the top corner, starting with A and the room or area. I also label the top of the box. This way, I can almost always find a label, even when they are stacked.

The notebook will be the record for these boxes, should you need to find anything. Box A has page 1 in the notebook. List the room at the top, then list all the contents in box A on that page. If you do need something, this will help you to find it quickly and easily.

I stored all our moving boxes, once packed, in our garage. One corner was for items that were moving with us, the other corner was for items for the big garage sale.

PLAN FOR THE SECOND PURGE

Think carefully about what you are keeping, and how it will be used when in a new place. It's also key to know that, no matter how much you purge and how ruthless you think you're being, if you're moving, there *will* be a second purge when you go to unpack!

I had 6 sets of dishes when we resized. My wedding china, my grandmother's china, my mother's china and three casual sets of dishes for 12. We did not put a dining room or nook in our home. We can seat 4 on our large, 10' island, eat on the patio if the weather is good, or eat sitting on the couch. So, I got rid of my wedding china, and packed up mom's and grandma's since I have a small longer term storage area for them.

Yet I *still* arrived in my new home with *three* sets of dishes, each serving 12. I shook my head at my own idiocy as I packed those up again to be donated. There was lots of purging as I unpacked and lots of self-talk that sounded like "what the hell was I thinking."

CHAPTER ACTION STEPS:

1. *Do you have a written plan and all the necessary supplies?*
2. *Have you had a family meeting and made agreements?*
3. *Make sure your staging spaces are ready for any stored items, and that your car is empty, ready to transport gifted or donated items!*

Chapter Eight

YOUR STUFF AND THE FOUR G'S

*W*hen I went through our own personal decluttering and resizing, every item was special to me. I was the person I had been helping all these years. My grandma had saved for 6 months to buy those Ginger sewing shears, she called them the "cadillac" of scissors. Now the shoe was on the other foot, and after years of helping others, I was now the one needing advice. And I learned a few things and created what I call the four Gs of decluttering for deciding what stays and goes.

Let's look at each category, ways to process and optional ways to use or manage these items.

GUILT

I will go right to the top of the emotional heap and start with family treasures.

Oh, the guilt!

You *must* keep Great Grandma Olive's tiny ceramic horse collection.

Really? I recall it at her house and loved playing with them all. They bought back fun memories. Can I visualize them in my head, or do I *need* them physically present to be happy? I don't even like horses.

This is the internal dialogue of guilt in your head. Get ready, because it is coming for you. *Hard.* And it will tug at your heartstrings, make you all mushy and melancholy, so get ready because *this is war*, I tell you.

Guilt Items are the ones I keep because they were special...to someone else, usually. Or they have extreme sentimental value. Like drawings that your kids did in the 1st grade. Tracings of their little hands. Grandma Coburn's casserole dish. Nana Grace's silver carving knife. Photos, memorabilia, tchotchkes, trinkets, jewelry and weird things like old eyeglasses and wallets.

At face value, they are maybe not anything special, but they belonged to someone special who is generally no longer with us. And this makes them very hard to part with.

In Chapter 6, I discussed letting go and mindset with the help of an exercise. At any time if you are struggling with that, feel free to revisit the exercise for some additional help. Let's look at some clever ways to approach these things.

My grandma Fran wasn't a fancy lady, but she acquired a silver-plated tea service. It was very pretty, but not valuable. I did not drink tea, it did not fit my décor, it was broken (the knob came off the teapot lid and couldn't really be fixed properly) and cumbersome. But it was Fran's, so I carted that sucker around for 10 years. At Christmas, I would make small flower arrangements in the sugar and cream bowls, but that was all. One day, I took this treasure and a few others of similar ilk, all cool but I was not attached to them, and I connected to many of my cousins by email with photos, saying these were things of our grandmother's, and who would ENJOY them, as I was not using them for enjoyment. I was surprised to get replies for every item, and I dropped some off, and mailed some others. And, like that, they were gone, and into the hands of others who were excited to own them! Win-win.

Guilt items can have special rules. I call it the strings-attached give. If I am a bit hesitant about something (usually a guilt item), I offer it to someone on the condition that if they ever don't want the item any longer, they will give it back to me first before just getting rid of the item. By then, I might be ok with it going elsewhere, but it is a bit of a safety net for any items with emotional connections. Yes, this only works if the recipient remembers or you trust them, so gift wisely.

Look at how you might repurpose guilt items. Can I use the china casserole dish for a fruit bowl? Let's be honest: if it is not pretty and pleasing to you in some way, why keep it? I have things I don't use often, but I use them in décor. That makes them useful to me in the long run, besides the sentimental value.

Can you take Grandma's sewing things and make a shadow box? My great grandma Olive did a lot of volunteering and when she passed, my grandma framed all her pins—Daughters of the Nile, Soroptimist, hospital name tags—on a velvet board that she framed. It was a pretty reminder of her, and her efforts, and we saw it all the time. A win-win again. An old gear from my father-in-law's farm that was all rusty and gross got scrubbed and sealed and is an interesting paperweight, watching me as I write this book.

GIVE

These are general items we all have. A friend has always admired those earrings or that bag. Maybe she would like them. If it has some value, is there a local charity that could use it? Would it be a gift someone else might enjoy and appreciate? Can I send it all to a local charity thrift store? This is generally the biggest group of stuff. If you are having a garage or estate sale, drop it all in that box, unless you specifically know of someone who might want it.

Be careful of the trap of gifting too many things to others, as this can really slow your process down. It takes time to contact them, ask them, get it to them, etc.

When considering items for GIVE, ask yourself the right questions.

- "Is it in good shape?"
- "Can or will I use it, or could someone else?"

- "If I did not own this, would I go out and buy it at full price?"
- "Does this add value to my life?"
- "Is this item making my life easier/harder?"
- "Is there someone who needs this more than me?"

These can help you move past the difficulty in parting with items.

When my mom passed, I received all her clothes. This was a massive undertaking. Three SUV's *full* of incredible designer clothes, shoes, and bags. She wore a bit bigger size than me, but her wardrobe was vast and had lots of variety.

I decided one day to invite 4 friends to my house who all knew my mom well. We grabbed a glass of wine and some snacks and sat in my family room for four hours. One by one, I pulled each item out of the bag and anyone interested would take it. If multiple ladies wanted one item, we set it aside and picked those in the end. As we went through everything, there were hysterical stories about what happened the night we went to a party and she wore this outfit. It was cathartic and felt good to share the things she really loved; she loved those clothes.

For years later, I would get texts from friends in a dress, top, or jacket of my mom's, "channeling Catherine today." That was an amazing gift!

As for the rest, I researched and found a local women's shelter and took two SUV loads to share with them. My mom would have approved!

GIVE items are great for garage or estate sales, gifting to others (even party style, like the clothes) donating to various charities or groups. It's a good feeling to know that things you can no longer use will benefit a good cause or help someone out; that's why this is my favorite category of things to get rid of.

GET SOME CASH

Some of mom's things that were very high end but no one fit or wanted, we sold online and then our family did something fun with the money. I knew my mom would approve of that because family time was very important to her. Getting cash for items is another good option.

Many items of value can be traded, sold, or consigned, so don't forget those methods. Price it to sell, as that is after all, the point of the exercise. Great options for goods and clothes can be eBay, Mercari, Offer up, Facebook marketplace or Poshmark.

The drawback here is you need to store the items until they are sold, so keep this in check or clutter will grow. Keep the items organized so you can retrieve and ship them quickly. And be sure to know the shipping costs so you are really making money when they sell. There are also lots of folks who will list for you for a percentage or fee, and consignment stores for clothing and furniture and décor items.

There are also local "freecycle pages" online and Buy Nothing on Facebook. Buy Nothing is an amazing international group that started in the town next to me to reduce landfill waste and help neighbors get to know each other. There are groups by geographic area, three in my small town alone. On Facebook, search "buy nothing" and the local groups will pop up. Choose the one you live in; you can only join one. You can give gifts or ask for items, no money or trades, just freely given.

My group is amazing. On a given day you will see anything from someone who made too much spaghetti offering dinner for 4 that night or a jar of jam someone tried a spoonful of and did not like. Everything you can imagine. All for free. You know that bottle of shampoo you bought that you hate the smell of? Buy Nothing will find it a home; it doesn't have to go in the trash. I am continually amazed by the odd and weird stuff offered, like the lid to a specific Tupperware bowl or a lid to a blender that is offered and several people comment to receive it. It's called the gifting economy, and it's here to stay.

Lots of young people just starting out ask for items you may have and not be using but didn't want to make the effort to find a home for. Be careful here too, because this can be time consuming, but for folks who like to know where their things are going, this can be a great way for them to feel okay about releasing things.

Read the rules; they vary from location to location. In my area, porch pickup is common – you set it out on an agreed upon day and the recipient picks it up. It's a fantastic option.

Garage Sales, Estate Sales and Auctions fall here too...hire an expert to manage the latter two. They know how to set it up and price it. Some will even take things off site to sell with several other families' items, and they have detailed systems for tracking your things. They know what is valuable and what is just from Target. They keep a percentage of the take, but they also set up prices, research, advertise, have repeat clients who follow them, sell, clean up and may even donate what's left.

There is a caveat in the category. Selling items, and even gifting, adds an extra layer and job to this already-involved process. You must research, price, photograph, list, figure out shipping, store the items so you can find them, find a box, ship them, deal with customers. For some, this is manageable. For others, this keeps them stuck. Consider this carefully and set timelines. If you list an item on Facebook Marketplace or eBay, make a commitment that if it is not sold in a specific timeline you lower the price, then in the next timeline if it is still not sold, you donate. This timeline should not exceed more than a few weeks in each area.

THE LAST G: GO AHEAD – STORE IT

If you are moving, this can be a must, like my mom's and grandma's china. It's my least favorite category, because it can spiral quickly with too many "I'm not sure" moments.

This category has limits. Without limits, it will linger. I recently unpacked 4 larger boxes from the resize move; it had been a few years. If there were 100 items in all 4 boxes, I bet I kept less than 20. If you GO ahead and pack it, and don't miss it in 1 year, or even 6 months, do you even need to open it and look through it? We both know the answer to that!

A friend admitted to me just last week she had a dozen boxes that she had not opened in 15 years. So, she tossed them, and was DONE. So freeing! But I know not everyone can do that.

Set limits, mark the calendar, and go through any Go-ahead items on pre-set dates.

CHAPTER ACTION STEPS:

1. *Who in your family or friend circle might be candidates for some of your "guilt" items?*
2. *If you are having a sale, when? Mark the date on the calendar or work on it, or find a person to manage it.*
3. *What system will you set up to manage the donated or gifted items quickly, and any items to be stored?*

Chapter Nine

SENTIMENTALITY AND THE WEIRD STUFF THAT SLOWS US DOWN

I am a very sentimental person, both about things and people. I think that was ingrained by my Grandma with whom I spent so much time growing up, and to whom I was so close.

My mom (daughter of this same grandma) was not terribly sentimental. Maybe about people, never about things. If they did not have a purpose or make her home lovely, out they went, and fast. Often things I had carted home from my grandma's would just disappear when I was not home. We had a large home and lots of storage, but that didn't matter. Not functional or useful? Out you go.

When I began my purge, I had so many sentimental items. I realize that I can come across in my writing as if my position were "toss it, gift it, get rid of it, but don't keep it," but that is really not the case. I help people resize, which is a somewhat ruthless activity. But I also know that there are things that serve no purpose or use that many of us simply cannot part with. It's up to you to make the final decision.

I have helped many people through this very process who, after decades of collecting and living life, did *not* want to declutter, or leave their home. There is a deep and heavy sadness to that kind of move, no matter how fun you try to make it.

When my sweet grandma left her home of roughly 45 years, I tried to encourage her that her new place was *so cute*. And it was, and maybe we could paint some walls her favorite blue, or arrange her artwork just so. She tried to be chipper about it, but she was sad. Even though she agreed to move, she only did so because she was being pushed to.

Every time I have done this, I have watched the clash between the family member who is moving and the family members who are trying to help, often with some anger or frustration that the moving family member is not "trying" hard enough.

They are trying. Trying to keep it together. Trying not to cry and feel overwhelmed, or even bullied. And they can often retreat as a result and do nothing. So, when I say "think very carefully about these items" or "really consider your mindset," I mean that in a way that is putting YOU in a power position. YOU are making these choices, for you. You are not being forced.

By all means, you can keep what you want and need, but that can become a very slippery slope, super quickly. In a best-case scenario, anyone resizing would be a little ruthless, but I realize all are not ready for such a dramatic step. Maybe it will take you a few tries. Maybe you will keep more or less than others. Maybe you will go nuts and declutter like a boss. Bottom line: I am here to share what has worked for me and the folks I have helped. You do you!

There are lots of personal items that can be very challenging to figure out how to save, preserve, and store. These can be the things that really slow you down, so I want to look at ways to handle some of the more sentimental items.

Before you begin the sentimental item purge, you may want to revisit the mindset exercise in chapter 6 to help you in processing these items.

I did a very informal survey of a friend group, and asked, "What are the things that are hard for you to part with, decide what to do with, or use?" Overwhelmingly I got the same answers, so I am dedicating this chapter to them.

But again: ***do what works for you!***

Be mindful of the trap of waiting to process some of these things later, but if it is truly what you need, you will know that. Many of the comments were that people were keeping the items that were special to someone else, but not to them. Because of their love for the person who owned the item, they keep it, not wanting to dishonor them. Some said it felt "heavy" to keep the items. Some keep things because they had little or nothing as kids (for many reasons, from poverty to parents who were chaotic or irresponsible) and many referenced how hard it was to get rid of things from their depression-era parents or grandparents, who often went without or saved for what seemed like an eternity to buy something we consider no big deal. It was both familiar and comforting to hear that from so many others.

When we can find ways to use, share, or incorporate these special items into daily life, that's a win. If we love them, they should not be in the back of a closet. Many times, I have come across things like this that were stored for "later." Often, they were ruined in storage, only to be thrown out. Water, pests, rodents, heat, etc. Storing things long term needs special consideration in order to preserve the item's integrity. So if you choose to store, store well! It's heartbreaking when someone opens a box of treasured items to find them moldy, covered in mouse poop, and ruined.

Keep in mind, anything stored in most attics or basements are not temperature-controlled, and can suffer the consequences. Things stored in outdoor sheds, or other uncontrolled environments begin rotting the minute you leave them there. They are almost destined to become trash, just very slowly. I personally think that is far more devastating than just gifting them to begin with.

Helping others in this process, especially when the person did not choose this for themselves 100% willingly, is an eye opening and life changing experience. It's given me clarity about what's really important in life, and what kind of mess I want to leave my child/family for later in my life, whether an estate or a needed resize. I'm choosing to take care of my own business, my own way, on my own terms. It's a choice each of us GETS to make, and it dramatically impacts those you leave behind or those who are helping in the process.

Let's also address money. For some people, losing money means they will keep an item. I am going to ask you to look at this in a very different light. Think about the things we buy. Many are purchased to be consumed (food) or used til no longer good (clothes, linens) and for a purpose that also leaves the item in decline (an older car). We buy items with the intent of consumption, and the use of those items is part of the cost. Very rarely do we buy *things* that are investments.

About a year ago, my husband bought a very expensive wool jacket. It was too hot to wear where we live, and he only wore it once a year on a trip to Montana. In the last year, he lost a fair bit of weight. The jacket no longer fit, and was too warm to wear where we lived. He wanted to keep it because of the cost. We just kept moving it around. Finally, I suggested we list it on eBay for $100 less than we paid. The proceeds were still a lot of money. We sold it, and he was able to pick out a new jacket that fit and was a more appropriate weight for our climate. For me, that was a win.

All our clutter used to be money. It took our time to make that money. It took our energy. For years many of us have been spending time, money, and energy to create a mess to be cleaned up later. That saying alone helps me to put things down I might buy if I don't really need them.

For many, the idea of donating eases the stress of giving things up. For others, the idea of sorting all this stuff out and trying to find homes is more distressing than getting a dumpster delivered.

For this reason, you must evaluate what will work best for you! What will keep you moving forward?

PAPER EPHEMERA:

This is a huge category. *Huge*. Kids artwork and school stuff, greeting cards and letters, old gift boxes, photos, scrapbooks, diplomas, funeral and wedding programs, birth and wedding announcements, yearbooks, books, I could go on for days here!

Years ago, my mother-in-law made a large box for each of her three grown kids. It was filled with report cards, childhood art and pottery, baby clothes, baby books, sports, fair and dance awards. To be honest, my mother-in-law couldn't toss it, so she did the next best thing, she gave it to the original owners. Now it was theirs to manage, keep, toss or save. Smart move.

Photos and photo albums, newspaper clippings, and odd papers that "seem" important. These can really put the brakes on progress. In many cases, I have made a photo tub where we corral all these items to deal with separately, sometimes at a later date.

Recently, I have been scanning all things possible. It is amazing how much space papers take up. I started with my 7 years of old tax and household records. I had 12 bins, each about 15 x 18 x 18". I went one by one, and I first went through and removed all the staples, neatened the piles then fed them through a scanner feeder. I did not organize the records by type, if I must go back and look, I will just look through. I do this now monthly and scan all records by type and file by month and year. This freed up a ton of storage space.

You can scan photos, greeting cards, kids' art, letters, yearbooks and more. Do you save magazines? Scan the pages you want or take a snapshot with your smartphone. There are so many ways to save ideas now that there is no good reason to have boxes, bins, and stacks around.

You can also make photo bins for your family. My grandma did this when she was resizing, any pictures of each kid went in their box, family photos got divided up. Photo books are also popular and are made easily online.

I purchased a fantastic scanner, the Fujitsu ScanSnap 1600. Not going to lie, I bought one for home and one for work. They are easy, fast, don't jam, and have a photo setting and album mode. I have thousands of family photos up to 100 plus years old. Thanks Fran! I haven't started yet, but it is a project on my list to scan them all. Then I will divvy up the originals to share with relatives, along with proving a thumb drive of all the digital images. Merry Christmas and Happy Hanukkah to you all!

Bonus, if you have a large scanning project, you can buy a scanner and resell when complete if you feel you don't need a scanner long term.

I often hear people say something along these lines: "Well, every now and then I like to pull them out and go through them" with regard to old letters, greeting cards, photos, photo albums. But guess what? When did you do that last? And, if you scan, you still can print, and you can share. It's just a format change, and a mindset change. You still have them, just not taking up space.

Frame some of those photos if they are that special. Hang some of that art. Frame a special piece your kid made and hang it in a prominent space (they will feel soooo honored! Trust me!) Do something with these treasures other than stuff them in a box in your attic, garage, or basement where at some point they most likely will be peed on by mice!

PARENTS AND GRANDPARENTS:

Anything and everything in this category circles back to the GUILT section of the 4 G's. This came up from almost everyone I surveyed. "It was my parents' or grandparents' item and I love them so much I can't bear to part with it" was pretty much the refrain. Along with "even though it's not special to me." Ugh. The knife to the heart. What to do? It really does feel like a betrayal!

The category is also large and can cover everything from dishes, china, glassware, artwork, old fur coats, personal effects like eyeglasses, professional tools from their life, jewelry or watches, furniture pieces, collectibles, and so much more.

This category takes a lot more effort than most, so feel free to save it for last, but I suggest processing it as you go. I firmly believe that if you don't love it, it should be someone else's. Guilt keeps are never fun. So, as you go through these items, even gathering them all in one space, where you can see how much you really have, can help you cut things down.

When you look at the whole, grab out the things that have special meaning to you. The vase your grandma always used, or the wooden nut bowl that held the nutcracker and picks that she only used at Christmas because "nuts are so expensive." Set those aside.

Then do round two. Are there any things that you could repurpose? A bowl that you could use as part of a display, or incorporate into daily use? A basket or container that could hold art supplies, snacks for the kids, pet toys. Can you make the items into something else? Something useful or even decorative and crafty (P.S. you can hire the crafter if you are not crafty!)? More on that later in this chapter.

Any sort of container, glasses, casserole dishes or bowls can be used to store everyday items. Glasses or small containers can be used for makeup brushes, eye pencils, art suppliers, pens, so many things.

If you have beautiful dishes or china, use it daily. That's right, make it your daily driver! My grandma would love to know that I use her beautiful things every day. Yes, something might break, it could happen, but using your things is worth that risk. It could be damaged in storage too.

Many friends mentioned multiples, for example china sets or dishes from moms. Grandmas, maybe even great grandmas and more. My rule of thumb here is to pick your favorite. As mentioned previously, I had 6 complete sets of dishes and china, complete with serving dishes, before resizing. *Six*. I could serve 12 to 20 with each in most cases. I narrowed it down to two: my mom's Franciscan Apple pattern, and a very old Prussian bone china set my grandma had given me that was her mom's before her. And the rest I sold or gifted, and felt pretty good about.

Sentimental items are a little more challenging, but there are many ways to reuse them and give them a place of honor. Or a little time; sometimes it's just too soon. When everyday items can be made useful or decorative, that changes them from clutter to something that brings joy.

For example, my husband's granny had so many beautiful handkerchiefs. Totally by happenstance, I found a woman on Etsy who folded and pinned them into beautiful vintage dresses about the size of a barbie dress. We sent them all off, and when they returned, we placed them in shadow boxes and all the girls in the family got one. The hankie itself would have been clutter, but the dress hangs in my office and I enjoy it daily! This also can be a great family gift. It's a fun way to display a cherished person's things and be reminded of them.

HOUSEHOLD ITEMS:

Whether sentimental or not, these items are generally larger, and take up more space. VCR/ Cassette tapes/ CD collections, collections of any kind, artwork or crafted items like Afghans/quilts, fabric and arts/crafts supplies, bags and boxes (yes, this is a real problem for my friends!).

I often loathe new technology. Pandora? Why, I have all these great CD's! But guess what, I ditched all 400 of them because they are online, and most of them are *free*. Yes, you can also purchase a plan very inexpensively, but it's not required. And now Spotify is my go-to for all things music. I took all the old family movies and sent them to a place that put them on DVD's....Christmas was covered that year....you get a DVD, and you get a DVD. You get the idea. And, everyone loved it!

Collections are tricky. I have had some. And usually, I got tired of them or my taste changed, or my space changed. Some got sold. Some got gifted. I kept only the most treasured.

One friend surveyed said: "My collection of beanie babies! (I keep saying I will sell some but when I see the resale value I feel they mean more to me than what I would earn from selling them so I continue to keep all 200 even though we don't have room to put them all out)."

I thought about this for a while. 200 of *anything* is a lot. Storing them properly, keeping moisture, pests and rodents away, deciding where to put them, all of that takes time and effort that could be spent on other things. Let's say the collection is valued at $2000. Meaning that was the cost to acquire. For many, losing money is not ok, so they keep things instead of selling at a loss. But consider this:if they are in boxes, are you enjoying them? If they are packed up, are they useful or in the way? How much did you spend on storage tubs to keep them in? If they have outlived their purpose for bringing you joy, is it time for them to move on?

Let's say you sell them for $1000. Many would jump to "well, I just lost a grand." But I see it differently. I just sold some things that were not bringing me joy, and while I did not get my financial investment back (when do we ever?), I now have $1000 AND a big area of free space I did not have before. I can take that money and go on a weekend trip with the hubs, buy something we have been wanting, upgrade something in the house, put it in savings or any other number of positive things you can make out of that sale! It's about mindset.

Artwork, paintings and the like can be tricky. My grandma was a semi-professional painter and entered juried competitions often, winning many ribbons and prizes. She was also prolific. There were maybe 100 framed pieces when she died, and not 100 family members. Even when I took just the ones I loved, that was still a dozen. Then there were the ones I took because no one else wanted them and they were so pretty. Now I had 2 dozen. And, I had no place to hang them for the most part. Eventually I gifted them to family and close friends, even to the new owners of her longtime home, who were *thrilled* to have one.

Afghans/quilts and the like are always tough, and usually have a lot of sentiment attached. Recently I went through an entire tall moving box of blankets. There had to be 20 quilts, afghans and other blankets. I looked carefully and took my time to choose the ONE that really spoke to me. My sister-in-law inherited all the quilts and toppers that had been stored by her grandmother and great grandmother. A gifted seamstress, she made quilts out of them for EACH of the siblings' kids. Useful and kept in good condition to enjoy for years to come. And a super thoughtful gift (again, this can be hired out).

Arts/Crafts/Fabric supplies. So, my friends appear to be crafty. I too have a lot of art supplies. A lot. Like I might be able to open a small art supply store. I collect craft things like old rhinestone jewelry, and other oddities. And they can cause clutter so fast. So, I keep them organized. It is so much easier to find and retrieve smaller items so I always try to keep them together. Bins, boxes, decorative containers, rolling storage carts with drawers: these and a label maker, like things together, will keep you from losing your mind. I know that my artistic interests change over time. So once a year, I do a quick sort and purge. Local schools and teachers LOVE your old craft castoffs. If year after year you keep seeing the same items and they are not getting used, maybe you need to be a bit more ruthless!

BAGS/BOXES AND ODD STUFF:

There are weird items we all have.

I was helping a dear friend move once. She had a very large kitchen with loads of cabinetry. We opened up a big cabinet and it was full of... empty Nordstrom boxes. Now these are nice gift boxes. Not like the flat white ones you get at Target. And she had nested them all together. I'm not exaggerating when I say there might have been 40. As I laughed so hard I might have peed a little, my friend said, "But I might need a gift box, you never know, and these are really nice." We still laugh about that.

That same friend's daughter told me in my survey, "bags of grocery bags" were her problem. Right? Whether paper, plastic or reusable, we all have them. Ways to limit things like this is to have a container. I have a wall mounted container in a cabinet that holds plastic bags. When it is full, I either recycle them and start over, keeping a few, or drop them at my local food bank which loves getting them. Same with paper bags. I have a bin, when full, I donate or recycle. So, for any of these types of items, create a container for them, label it and when full, choose the appropriate action.

I have some very cool stacking plastic drawers in the corner of my small closet. There are three, they take up maybe 12 x 18 x 24". They are my "donation" drawers. I place items there that are to be donated to the local thrift store. When the drawers are full, I grab a bag from my bag bin, and I place the bag or bags in my car so I can drop them off. Works like a charm.

CLOTHING:

This is the second most mentioned category in my survey. And what are people keeping? Vintage clothes that were their mom's/grandma's or beautiful clothes they no longer fit in and cannot seem to part with. One single friend admitted that every closet in her 3 bedroom home was *full* of clothes she couldn't wear.

Vintage clothes are so fun. My seamstress grandma made so many beautiful clothes. And I have a few. One dress in particular we had altered, and my daughter wore it to a dance. It was a dress my grandma had made to go to dances with my grandpa. It was so pretty and my daughter was floored by the insane amount of compliments she got, as it was not like everyone else's. So, alter it and wear it!

Clothes that don't fit are tricky. Or, clothes that were *very* expensive, like cocktail gowns and the like. I like to joke about my expensive jeans habit and cost per wear. Let's be honest, it's for shoes too. If the jeans are $250 and I wear them for three years 1 day a week that is only $1.60 per wear, and while I really never do the math, you get the idea. And I will wear them much more than 3 years because the quality is so good.

I had a stunning black and pink harlequin pattern wool blazer, double breasted, that I bought at Nordstrom in the early 1990's. I used to wear it with my black cat suit (remember those? Basically, a unitard for skinny girls) and I thought I was the shizzle. It was hands-down, at the time, the most expensive thing I ever bought, just shy of $200.00. So, I kept it. Almost 30 years later, I decided I could finally let it go. I wore the hell out of it in the early 1990's. So, the cost per wear worked out, but emotionally it was hard to part with, even though I could not have fit into it any longer. I still hung on. I was more attached to the memories of it, and the people I wore it with and the places we went and experiences we had. When I realized that, it was easy to set it free.

We are fortunate to have lots of options for these clothes to recoup some of the costs: resale shops, online platforms, online resellers. So, what a treat would it be to rid yourself of some of the items (at a minimum) and then buy yourself something that makes you feel amazing, that fits, that you can wear and enjoy? Part of the price of any item is enjoyment of use. And you generally got that out of it, right?

I used to go to a lot of formal events and, you know, you "can't" wear the same dress twice in the same crowd, right? Well, now I rent my dresses. That's right. *Rent.* Last year I went to a 3 day Pakistani wedding extravaganza (seriously, it was so epic!). Rent the Runway to the rescue! I had 4 dresses that cost me about $150 total to rent, and each one was a major designer dress worth $1500 or more. I felt like a damn princess. I can't wait to do it again! After the wedding, I mailed them back, and that was that!

THE REST OF THE WEIRD STUFF:

Let's face it, there are many items in a home that cause people to struggle about what to do with them. They don't have a specific use, more of a memory or sentimentality that makes it hard to part with. My informal survey identified many of these and I will address them here.

I have turned many things that did not have a use for me (my grandma's handkerchiefs or jewelry for instance) into something cool, useful, or decorative that I can enjoy! Spend an hour surfing crafty sites like Etsy and Pinterest and you will have so many ideas. Or, google "what can I do with old _____?" The ideas will be endless. This list of these odd items is long, so let's dive in.

Have old tee shirts or clothes made into a tee shirt quilt. There can be a theme, or it can be random. Tee shirts can also be framed and displayed like art.

Smaller personal items like pocket knives—my father-in-law must have had 50 of them—that would make a fantastic display and reminder of him.

You can also have old clothes or furs made into teddy bears or throw pillows. This is especially nice for grandkids if a grandparent has passed. Many seamstresses offer this service. Also check Etsy.com to see if any sellers there can make them for you.

If you are crafty, check out Pinterest. You can learn a new way to repurpose anything on this fun social media site.

Example: I have a lot of doilies. Type doilies into the search bar on Pinterest and viola, there you have 200 ways to use doilies, and I am sure one might be just perfect for you! Just try it. "Uses for old tee shirts," "vintage china crafts." It's a fun way to waste an afternoon scrolling, but seriously, some very great ideas there.

A fun idea for small things is shadow boxes. I personally love these, and they can be made as gifts. We have had pets all our lives. When they pass, they have a collar and leash, lots of photos, maybe a favorite toy. Why not make a shadowbox of pet items? Add some fun pictures of them. These can be fun art or a great and meaningful gift. My grandma was an incredible seamstress and pattern drafter. She made my wedding gown by hand, changing up the pattern, altering the back, sleeves, and skirt, and created a full skirt and train for the ceremony that then unsnapped under the lace from the bodice afterwards for the reception, leaving me with a pencil skirt gown that was much easier to dance and walk around in. Her sewing shears, some of her accessories like her pin cushion, scraps of fabric and old spools of her thread combined with a few photos would be a beautiful shadow box.

Use grandma's old teacups as little planters, plant small flowering plants and share on Mayday or Easter. Create mini flower arrangements, silk or fresh, for birthdays. If you are crafty, pour candles in the teacups. Search teacup crafts on Pinterest...it's a rabbit hole, use caution! And be realistic. Will you really try that craft that has so many steps and supplies needed or is there a simpler way? Many people just don't see things in a repurposed way, so Pinterest can be a great visual cue for folks on how to make seemingly useless items useful in daily life or décor.

Books can take up so much space, and as we age our eyes change and people tell me they still read but slower. They need to slow down the rate at which they buy new books so as to not overload.

I love a high shelf around the perimeter of a room for book storage. If you have a lot of books, custom-built ins can be a game changer. Custom because they can be done with adjustable shelves, and to any depth you want or need where buying them off the shelf they are standard pre-set size. We do a lot of custom casework in our builds and remodels and offices and bookcases are big. Clients tell us how many and what size books they have so we can design a system that works well for the book types they have. Anything custom will cost more, but it also is THE most effective and efficient way to store things. Built perfectly to an opening or height, it gives you the ability to use all the space!

I have my share of books, but I try to keep my physical collection to 100 or less as I really don't have the space for many more. I also happen to enjoy audio books, so I have a large Audible library. I am often guilty of buying the Audible book AND the paper book, usually off eBay if available. I do try to do a regular purge of my physical books so that they don't get out of control.

Have a party. That's right: *a party*.

My mom had so many beautiful things, and so many holiday decorations and items. I took a large box to a family gathering and everyone chose what they wanted. Sometimes it feels very different to gift things to people who knew and loved your loved one than donating to strangers. Or have a dessert night at your house and ask your friends over and let them choose some items.

This is akin to something called "Swedish Death Cleansing" and there are many great books on the topic. It's the brainchild of Margareta Magnussen who only recently coined the term with her book in 2017 "The Gentle Art of Swedish Death Cleaning: How to Free Yourself and Your Family From a Lifetime of Clutter." In practical terms, it's about organizing and decluttering your home to reduce the burden of sorting through belongings to decide what is significant. It can be undertaken at any life stage or age, but should be done sooner rather than later, before others must do it on your behalf.

Give personal items as gifts. Most of us have all the "stuff" we need. For years there was a small, old, beat to hell blue gas can at my in-laws house. I always loved it and told my mother-in-law. She had it up high with some pussy willow stems in it. One Christmas, I opened a gift and there was the can. I was over the moon! It was the perfect gift for me. Giving it away got it out of her house, put it in the hands of someone who appreciated it and would treasure it, and it cost her nothing.

When it comes to the sentimental stuff, many people will slow down, be more resistant and face indecision. I am not here to tell you it has to go. I am here to encourage you to fully consider WHY you are hanging on to it. If this section takes you a little more time, so be it. This is a space that everyone reacts to differently. And for some it can take some time to come around scanning things instead of keeping them and the like. Don't be too hard on yourself if you are having trouble parting, just keep moving and you will get there.

CHAPTER ACTION STEPS:

1. *If you have a large number of sentimental items, can you break them into smaller groupings, or set aside to do all at one time?*
2. *What sentimental items do you have that can be creatively repurposed for you or others or given as gifts?*
3. *What creative ways can you use or display some of the problem items so they are a feature of your home and you can enjoy them?*

Chapter Ten

WHAT TO KNOW ABOUT SMALLER LIVING

*W*hen I started as a home builder, everyone wanted the same thing. Homes needed to have a formal living room *and* a family room. A formal dining room *and* an eat-in kitchen, and the average home in my market was about 1800 square feet. That meant a lot of small, choppy rooms. It evolved to more of a great room style, losing the formal living room but keeping the dining room *and* nook.

Now, we see less and less formal spaces, but still a designated dining area. In my market, big homes still rule; 2500 square feet is now considered the bare minimum. When I began building, I always held the belief that a smaller, well-appointed home was far superior to a larger home with few features or amenities. But the market rules, so I have built my share of "drywall palaces" and "McMansions" that have zero character but nice countertops and cabinets and not much else to offer but square footage.

Smaller homes like mine are often referred to as "jewel box" homes, as they have all the features of a large home, and *more*. More built-ins, more details, higher end finishes and features, all of which add to the enjoyment of a space.

According to Investopedia.com the median single-family home in the US is 2532 square feet in 2021. In 1970 it was 1500 square feet, and in 1950 was 983 square feet.[1]

Smaller homes require a lot more thought in design and layout to function well than do larger homes. They take more preparation and planning. If you're planning to move, build or remodel, there is a lot to consider before choosing that resized home.

I always encourage people to consider what spaces or rooms or features they require in their home. Do you need an office, a sewing room, a guest room? Assigned places for your cat box, dog dishes, the Roomba? Think about all the things in your house. I encourage people to walk through each room and look for these items. They'll pop out immediately. Make a list of all those things. Then, make a master list of all the things that you need to consider.

Sarah Susanka is an architect and the author of a groundbreaking book series called "The Not So Big House." I am a huge fan, and she has many books on the topic of living smaller along with designs and remodeling advice. Her website is www.susanka.com.

If you are not moving, or are a renter, perhaps an interior designer can help you with a space plan or space modification? Space planning is a life saver and it shows you options for using your space in the best way possible. I recently tried this for a small space and it was amazing. I like to think I am pretty good at this but the options my designer came up with were nothing at all I would have ever thought of and they made the space feel so much bigger and well laid out. Worth every cent.

There are some great free options too; some of these programs have a bit of a learning curve but can be fun to use and helpful to be able to reconfigure spaces easily! Sketchup has a free version, Floorplanner, and IKEA makes an app called IKEA place app. All are great ways to DIY at no cost.

Storage. Where will you store things? If you're keeping china, and you don't have a dining room, where will that go? No matter how much we declutter, we will still need storage.

My family are sort of nomads: the longest we have lived anywhere is 12 years, and the shortest is 2 years. The last 3 homes have had dedicated walk-in storage rooms that were heated. Not fancy, concrete floor and taped drywall with a simple light. When you look at the cost and inconvenience of a storage unit, the fees, insurance, going there...it makes sense to create storage space, if needed, in your home or garage.

If you have items that you're keeping for a little bit longer term to see if you need them or they're just sentimental items you can't part with, where will they go? Make a list of all the things that are going to go into the house and how they will be managed. Mark your calendar to follow up on these items.

Next, look at your current furnishings. This scale is very important in any design, but in a smaller home scale is critical. There are furniture stores that specialize in smaller scale goods; search them out. A large sofa that fit in my old 3400 square foot house was a little much for my now 1131 square foot house. It didn't allow for a convenient furniture layout. It took up most of the space and the style just wasn't what I was headed towards. So that item was sold and replaced with something new. Think about the scale.

One thing you can do is use a floor plan and furniture templates to draw out the space and lay the furniture templates out to see if what you have will fit or if you need to make some new purchases or adjustments. Knowing that up-front will save you a lot of time and headache.

It's also important to think about room size. I know when we resized from 3400 square feet to 1131 square feet. I had to really think about the primary bedroom suite. Our old primary suite was very spacious. It held a king bed with large end tables. A dresser, a nice, overstuffed chair with a table and a reading lamp. We had a huge walk-in closet and a spacious five-piece primary suite bath. It was lovely. The primary suite bath included a makeup area and a large soaking tub.

In the new house, the bedroom was quite small and the bathroom even smaller. Five by eight for a primary suite, two sinks, a toilet, and a shower. A nice one, but still not super spacious. My walk-in closet was reduced from 10 by 12 to five by five. I had to think about where all those clothes would go that I couldn't fit in a five-by-five closet. In the summer, where would I store my winter clothes? In the winter, where would I store my summer clothes and shoes? I came up with an easy solution: a rolling rack that fit easily on the back wall of the garage and could be accessed as needed. It has a clear zippered cover and works great. I managed to swap things twice a year.

There is significant irony in my work. I recently realized that almost all the new builds the last several years have had primary suites larger than my *entire* home. Yep, that's right. And while they are lovely, I am perfectly happy living in this reduced size home!

Think about those sorts of things. Where will all the extras go? Where do you store the odd things like suitcases and other stuff like that. You want to make sure to design a space that accommodates all those things. In a small house, you must take the chance to maximize every space there is and figure out where you can sneak in storage. If you're building or remodeling, there can be a lot of opportunities to use wall cavities for storage space. I've seen cabinet companies that do toe-kick drawers (drawers that are built into the space between the baseboard and the bottom cabinets). They were very expensive. I'm not sure that the tradeoff is worth it. But yes, they do add extra storage and some people do want them.

Are there spaces where you could do a built-in wall cabinet or some sort of secret compartment? Those are great places to store small things like jewelry, all kinds of treasures. Walking through a house during framing is a great way to spot some of those and ask your contractor "Hey, what's going in that void?" The voids are often dedicated for things like ductwork, exhaust pipes, venting, heat supply and power. So not all spaces are fair game. You'll need to ask and get input.

You need to stay organized in a small home. And one way to do that is regular purging. So don't think that your decluttering is over! My rule is: when something comes in, something must go, and I stick to it well. Every now and then my cabinets and cupboards get a little overloaded and I must do a little bit of a clean out. It's how life works. Small details make huge impacts in smaller living. Drawer organizers and cabinet bins are game changers for keeping things tidy and neat and easy to find. There is a list at the end of the book under resources that will give you links to a lot of my favorite organizing products that really help convert spaces and customize them into what you need.

Think about the things no one likes to think about. What about a vault or a safe, valuable storage; if there are firearms in the home, are they stored safely? Hobbies, kids' gear? Kitchen trash and recycling (I hate looking at them and they are a trip hazard). The vacuum cleaner, mop and broom. Pet dishes. The list is endless.

Look at what you're currently housing and what's a current problem zone for you. Is it at the back door where the kids come in and just throw everything down? Maybe it's at the front door? Can you create a locker system or a storage system, their shoe bins, shoe drawers, anything to manage all of that? Coat racks, individual cubbies for each kid. That's a perfect example of managing things at the source right where kids come in. They can hang up their backpack, their coat, and put their shoes away. And then when things are ready for school the next day, they can be set in their storage zone so they're ready to go.

Those kinds of details really keep clutter at a minimum and everyone knows where their things are. No one ever seems to know where to put the dog dish, cat box or the Robot vacuum and charging station. If you plan ahead, that can really help you. I like to put cat boxes in cabinets or closets, and I even vent them with exhaust fans. Cats can sneak in a little cat door and do their thing. Food dishes can be put away that way too. Many cabinet companies make a pull-out lower drawer that has pet food dishes. You can have recesses or open spaces at the end of a bathroom vanity for a hamper so it's not sitting out in the end of the room. And in every kitchen I design, I make sure that there is a cabinet with a trash and recycle bin. I didn't spend all that time designing you a beautiful kitchen so you could have a $20 garbage can sitting at the end of your lovely new island.

Think about the storage options and how you might conceal or manage some of those things. Staying organized does require family participation so make sure that everyone in your home knows where their things belong; try to work with them to their organizing type so that they will participate. That is key to managing life in a smaller home.

CHAPTER ACTION STEPS:

1. *Is smaller living something you want to try out? How will you do that?*
2. *How much could you save by resizing, and what would, or could you do with that extra money?*
3. *If smaller living is not for you, what can you do to your current home to create less clutter and make it the best environment for you and your family?*

Chapter Eleven

SIMPLE SYSTEMS TO KEEP IT ALL GOING

*C*ongratulations! You've read through all the steps to begin your own decluttering and resizing process.

Are you ready? This is where the rubber meets the road. It's time to go back through and start the work.

Once your process is complete, you will need a plan to keep everything in order and avoid going back to overwhelm and clutter. That's where this last chapter comes in.

I have some simple rules about managing clutter to share, and there are loads and loads of books on the subject if you want more detailed systems.

Things move fast in a digital world, so I keep an updated list of my favorite organizing products and resources on my website to keep you on track: www.judygranleegates.com.

HERE ARE A FEW EXAMPLES:

www.organize365.com This is the Sunday Basket method and is a great plan for weekly review and management of problem items like bills, mail, school papers, returns.

www.banishbusinessclutter.com by Lydia Martin. This refers to business, but Lydia specializes in paper clutter. And that is the stuff that really gets out of hand and takes up so much space. Lydia offers courses and community to support you in a digital declutter, and I highly recommend her courses. They have really changed the way I manage paper, but I will be honest, paper is my kryptonite, and I still struggle with paper. Lydia uses scanners, apps and other methods to help manage the paper, and she is a genius at it. The things I learned were so simple, and so impactful.

Join a Facebook group that has to do with organization, decluttering or resizing. Or join several. Folks who are actively doing this on the daily will have great tips and solutions, and you can post photos or questions to the "hive mind" and get some really incredible answers, all for free! Just search by keyword on Facebook, join a few, and see which ones resonate.

Invest in a label maker. It sounds cliché and micro-managey...but it works. If people know where it goes, they will *usually* put it there. Try it. Label inside of drawers and cabinets, bins that go in drawers and cabinets... It really does make a difference. Not gonna lie, I have 3 label makers. One at home, at the office and at a cabin we have. We rent our cabin out when not there and the #1 comment from our guests about what they love after the space is that everything is labeled so they always know where to find it, and even more helpfully, where to put it back!

Use clear bins and boxes to corral similar items. People like me think the container store is heaven on earth (it is, I swoon there). I love organizing bins and containers; they make finding and storing things a breeze.

If new stuff comes in, something's gotta go. Purge regularly and donate promptly.

If you live in a smaller space, think about high bookshelves. Or floor-to-ceiling ones. I have a small office / art studio and around the top 15" of the room is a book shelf that holds all my books, of course displayed in ROY G BIV like all crazy organized folks (that is an acronym for the order of colors in a rainbow and an organizers dream... Red, Orange, Yellow, Green, Blue, Indigo, Violet). I smile every time I walk in.

Start a gift space. I know so many people who buy the perfect gift when they see it (me!) and can't find it when it's time to give the gift (hello, that used to be me!). Now I have a bin in a closet, and that is where they go. When I need the gift, I go grab it. It can be a bin, box, drawer, cabinet, whatever space you like.

To keep things moving out of the house, start a "donation" bin. Same concept, and when full, take it off to donate. I also do this with things that need to be returned to others, like the casserole dish my friend brought to dinner, or a left-behind toy of a niece or nephew. This way you know right where it is and can grab it to return on the next meet-up.

Add furniture pieces that offer storage such as small ottomans, built in cabinetry perfect for the shape and size of a specific space. Cabinets to the ceiling for extra storage on top. Cabinet roll trays under the sinks in the kitchen and bath. You will likely have to modify or hire a carpenter to miss the drainpipe, but when you need something, roll the tray out and grab it, no more unloading the entire cabinet. Same with those obnoxious over-the-refrigerator cabinets that are so deep. You need a step ladder to get in there anyway; add a roll tray for ease in retrieving those things.

Hang art and décor wall to wall or floor to ceiling for high visual impact!

Use drawer organizers to keep similar things together, neat and tidy.

Hooks or shoe organizers on the backs of doors create extra hanging and small item storage.

Pretty storage for the win. Decorative bins. Boxes, baskets, jars, containers make storing small unruly things much easier. Search out some you like to keep all sorts of things in. A great way to keep tidy and add color. You can label them, add decorative tags, etc.

Curate boards on Pinterest.com to help inspire you. You can search by space, by project, you name it. It's my favorite social media site. Now I just have closet envy, but I can act on that. On most platforms, I have travel- or experience-envy, which can't be solved as quickly.

It's time to sit back and enjoy the peace and harmony you have created. Spend more time seeing and doing than cleaning and finding, adventuring and exploring than yard work and house chores. Making new memories to add to the old, cherished ones.

My hope for you, dear reader, is that you now see a path to a simpler, richer life, all because of how you manage your stuff. It's been a game-changer in my family, and I can't wait to hear how it has impacted you!

CHAPTER ACTION STEPS:

1. *What actions have you taken to understand other family members' organizing style?*
2. *What organizational tips will you implement to keep things orderly?*
3. *How often will you follow up or check-in for ongoing decluttering?*

ACKNOWLEDGMENTS

This book would likely not exist without the support of my husband and business partner, Joe, who entertains many of my half-baked ideas, including building an 1100 square foot home, or my publisher, Sierra Melcher for working with me so diligently to distill my concept. My research assistant Greer Gates saved me a lot of time, and also provided incredible tech support when needed. Dr. Adrienne MacIain Ph.D. inspired and energized my creativity when the faucet ran dry.

Outline review meetings with Shabnam Ananda, Jessica Goldmuntz Stokes, and Frances Trejo-Ley. These ladies gave me incredible input that really helped define my message and focus when I was waffling. Thank you for the time and energy to help me create this book and see my message more clearly.

Special thanks to Maya Amaele Liebermann for beta reading and content editing and development, along with title and chapter content, and Christina Hanson for beta reading, content editing, and development. Both offered excellent help, reading the entire manuscript, and gave incredibly rich and wildly detailed feedback to make the book the best it could be.

To so many friends and my family who encouraged me on this daunting task, and supported me to make this book a reality. Many of you commented on research posts, gave important feedback on concepts, and helped me narrow down specifics by answering simple questions that would benefit my readers.

Kirsten Friedman, LMHC, Certified Psychodramatist, TEP, Certified Therapist - Internal Family Systems for her help with IFT and mindset change about letting go!

My silent mentors: Mel Robbins, Jon Acuff, Sara Dean, and Jessica Butts (not really silent), who inspired and encouraged me countless times with pep talks, subject matter I needed to hear, and helped me expand my horizons to achieve this goal. Three of you are strangers, and one a friend, who have always felt like a best friend giving me personalized advice. Thank you for all you put out into the world to support and encourage.

To you, who are reading this book. I wrote this to help folks avoid the pressure of a "forced" resize, and enjoy its many benefits earlier in life. Thank you for your purchase and trust.

ABOUT THE AUTHOR

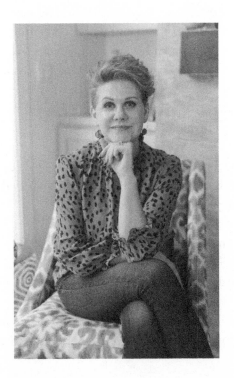

Judy Granlee-Gates began her first job at age 7 in her mom's hair salon, organizing the hair color bottles each week. She now organizes "for fun" with creative solutions and helping others with their projects large and small.

She is a professional problem solver in all environments, who helps overwhelmed clutter bugs create beautiful and peaceful environments letting go of clutter and taming chaos. She teaches people how to change their mindset and stop letting their things control them. With step-by-step guidance, she helps you declutter and resize your belongings and home to live a richer and fuller life with greater freedom: financial, emotional and time.

A fourth-generation small business owner and multi vocational woman, Judy Granlee-Gates has worked in Residential Construction since 1989 and strives for continual improvement in her processes and has helped hundreds of clients resize their homes. She is a driven problem solver and uses her organizational skills to benefit her customer's experience. She is an award-winning custom home builder and remodeler; dozens of her projects have been recognized on local, state and national levels and her company received a Pacesetter Award from Custom Home Magazine for outstanding customer experience. Judy utilizes her degree in Education, Training and Development to take her customers through the homebuilding and remodeling process with confidence, fun and outstanding results.

She is a construction industry blogger, owns a successful and popular Vacation Home Rental in Central Washington, an avid note writer and sender, an active philanthropist, and artist.

Judy is the parent of a grown "singleton" and lives in Western Washington State with her husband and pets.

linktr.ee/judygranleegates

Please visit Judy's website, **www.judygranleegates.com** for a free download plus links to her Facebook Community, other resources, and helpful tips.

instagram.com/decultterandresize

amazon.com/author/Judy-Granlee-Gates

THANK YOU

If you found this book helpful, I would greatly appreciate a simple review on **Amazon** at **amzn.to/3XMfWr9** or **GoodReads.**

ALSO BY JUDY GRANLEE-GATES

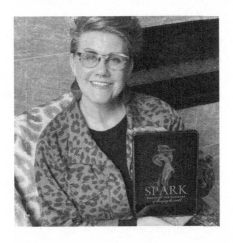

SPARK: Women in the Business of Changing the World
(Red Thread Publishing, 2022).

The world needs YOUR SPARK!

This collection of powerful voices and relatable experiences of women from around the world is a celebration of the extraordinary impact that ordinary women, women like you, can have when they show up and shine in their full, ***unapologetic authority.***

• What could YOU accomplish if you tuned in and owned your own brilliant light?

• What is YOUR gift for the world?

Regardless of where you live or how you grew up, you can change the world when you let your spark blaze!♥

May these stories transform and inspire you to unleash your own contagious spark within your life, in your community, and across the globe.

Authors hail from Australia, Morrocco, the United States, Colombia, the UK & beyond! These women share how they are making it their business to change the world, through career, purpose-driven & mission-based work of all kinds.

This book will not only INSPIRE but also TRANSFORM you!

Get your copy now! For a limited time at this unbeatable price.

✓ All royalties from this book are donated to the Red Thread Publishing's *First-Time Female Author fund*, to accomplish the mission of supporting 10,000 women to become successful published authors, entrepreneurs & thought leaders! With the purchase of this book, you are making that dream a reality for one more woman & changing the world. Thank you.

Do you want to become an author?

* Submit to the *First-Time Female Author Anthology* to become an author. https://forms.gle/miA4XqGS26QyT5T96

ABOUT THE PUBLISHER

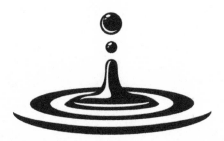

Red Thread Publishing is an all-female publishing company on a mission to support 10,000 women to become successful published authors and thought leaders. Through the transformative work of writing & telling our stories we are not only changed as individuals, but we are also changing the global narrative & thus the world.

www.redthreadbooks.com

 facebook.com/redthreadpublishing
 instagram.com/redthreadbooks

NOTES

2. LITTLE GHOSTS AND THEIR INCREDIBLY LOUD VOICES

1. Fees based on Kitsap County Washington Department of Community Development

3. TOUGH LOVE ON TIDYING UP

1. https://www.garageliving.com/blog/home-garage-stats
2. https://pickupplease.org/7-organization-stats/
3. Gamblin, A. 2018, 11 January, "It's science: Clutter can actually give you anxiety," Mother.Ly https://www.mother.ly/home/its-science-clutter-can-actually-give-you-anxiety/
4. Biggs, C. 2017, 29 June, "Study Reveals The Most Common Items that Go Missing at Home," www.apartmenttherapy.com, https://www.apartmenttherapy.com/study-reveals-the-most-common-items-that-go-missing-at-home-246906
5. Decluttr, 2015, 13 January, "Survey Finds 54 Percent of Americans are Overwhelmed with Clutter and Don't Know What to Do With It," www.prnewswire.com, https://www.prnewswire.com/news-releases/survey-finds-54-percent-of-americans-are-overwhelmed-with-clutter-and-dont-know-what-to-do-with-it-300019518.html
6. The Cleaning Authority, 2015 15 March, "Ready to Spring Clean? The Cleaning Authority® Says Start by De-cluttering," www.prnewswire.com, https://www.prnewswire.com/news-releases/ready-to-spring-clean-the-cleaning-authority-says-start-by-de-cluttering-300053707.html

5. AMERICA, LAND OF THE STORAGE UNITS

1. Harris, A, 2021 27 January, "US Self Storage Statistics," www.sparefoot.com, https://www.sparefoot.com/self-storage/news/1432-self-storage-industry-statistics/
2. https://www.neighbor.com/storage-blog/self-storage-industry-statistics/

7. YOUR BLUEPRINT FOR SUCCESS

1. P., K 2021 23 February "average Cost of Clothing Per Month Will Surprise You", www.creditdonkey.com, https://www.creditdonkey.com/average-cost-clothing-per-month.html
2. P., K 2021 23 February "average Cost of Clothing Per Month Will Surprise You", www.creditdonkey.com, https://www.creditdonkey.com/average-cost-clothing-per-month.html

10. WHAT TO KNOW ABOUT SMALLER LIVING

1. Smith, L, 2022 18 July "McMansions – A Closer Look at the Big House Trend", www.investopedia.com https://www.investopedia.com/articles/pf/07/mcmansion.asp

Made in the USA
Las Vegas, NV
31 January 2023

66573029R00062